Beginning Racquetball

Beginning Racquetball

SEVENTH EDITION

Cheryl Norton, Ed.D.

Southern Connecticut State University

James E. Bryant, Ed.D.

San Jose State University

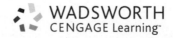

WADSWORTH
CENGAGE Learning

Australia • Brazil • Japan • Korea • Mexico • Singapore • Spain • United Kingdom • United States

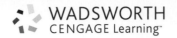

Beginning Racquetball, Seventh Edition
Cheryl Norton, Ed.D., James E. Bryant, Ed.D.

Publisher/Executive Editor: Yolanda Cossio

Print Buyer: Linda Hsu

Right Acquisition Director: Bob Kauser

Permissions Editors: Don Schlotman
(text & Image)

Production Manager: Matt Ballantyne

Acquisitions Editor: Laura Pople

Assistant Editor: Samantha Arvin

Developmental Editor: Liana Monari Sarkisian

Editorial Assistant/Associate: Kristina Chiapella

Technology Project Manager: Miriam Myers

Marketing Manager: Laura McGinn

Marketing Assistant/Associate: Elizabeth Wong

Art Director: John Walker

Manufacturing Manager: Marcia Locke

Production Service: PreMediaGlobal

Compositor: PreMediaGlobal

Cover Design: Betsy Bush

Cover Images: Masterfile

For product information and technology assistance, contact us at
Cengage Learning Customer & Sales Support, 1-800-354-9706

For permission to use material from this text or product,
submit all requests online at **cengage.com/permissions**
Further permissions questions can be emailed to
permissionrequest@cengage.com

Library of Congress Control Number: 2010935918

ISBN-13: 978-0-8400-4810-3

ISBN-10: 0-8400-4810-6

Wadsworth
10 Davis Drive
Belmont, CA 94002-3098
USA

Cengage Learning is a leading provider of customized learning solutions with office locations around the globe, including Singapore, the United Kingdom, Australia, Mexico, Brazil, and Japan. Locate your local office at:
international.cengage.com/region

Cengage Learning products are represented in Canada by Nelson Education, Ltd.

For your course and learning solutions, visit **academic.cengage.com**

Purchase any of our products at your local college store or at our preferred online store **www.cengagebrain.com**

Printed in the United States of America
1 2 3 4 5 6 7 14 13 12 11 10

Contents

The textbook serves as a guide to developing the physical and mental skills necessary to succeed in playing racquetball. The game is presented through photographs and figures, providing a visual concept of the game in order to assist in comprehension of how to play the game correctly.

"Points to Remember" and "Common Errors and How to Correct Them" highlight key information. As a tool for self-evaluation, a set of "Checkpoints" conclude each chapter. These are self-testing multiple choice questions designed to challenge and assist the student to focus on the most important aspects of the game.

We, as authors, confess to a feeling of confidence that, through the years of writing and experience, we have put together a truly quality book on racquetball that remains consistent to a great extent from the first edition through this seventh edition. What is of particular importance is that this edition continues to provide the quality reflected in the earlier editions while still presenting new information, changes, and new ways to understand the game. This edition includes a return to color figures, and changes in the "Checkpoints" questions provide a challenge to students. There is also an update of resources, particularly websites regarding racquetball. And, there is an extended effort to encourage students to be aware of the United States Racquetball Association (USRA) and its many outreaches to racquetball players. The USRA, in fact, provides the Racquetball Rules in the Appendix of the book, which enhances the learning experience for students. Although many of these content areas aren't new to this edition, they are promoted and enhanced as critical to the learning experience of students, and they enhance the instructor's ability to provide a full coverage of the game.

Cheryl Norton, Ed. D. and
James E. Bryant, Ed. D.

Acknowledgments

Contributions to this seventh edition of *Beginning Racquetball* are, in large part, a cumulative effect. Previous editions have been supported by creative ideas, suggestions by students, and efforts by reviewers, skilled photographers, and the production people who have digitally enhanced the figures, photos, and general appearance of the book. Our thanks go out to each and every one of these individuals who have contributed so much to the quality of the book.

Terrell Lloyd, who did most of the photography for this edition, and the most recent models Elda Shilts, Ve Le Dong, and Beau Batista deserve special credit. The Silicon Valley Athletic Club of San Jose, California, where the skill photographs were shot, deserve special recognition. Also, thanks go to the Sport Chalet of Antioch, California, for their assistance in supplying equipment to be photographed for the book. And lastly, the United States Racquetball Association (USRA) deserves very special recognition for its support and development of racquetball.

Cheryl Norton, Ed. D. and
James E. Bryant, Ed. D.

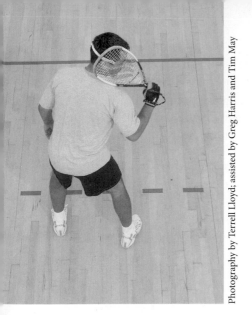

1

Court, Equipment, Safety, and Resources

Racquetball is played in an enclosed court using the four walls, floor, and ceiling as the playing surface. In areas where a four-wall court cannot be built, one- or three-wall racquetball may be played. The rules and strategy for these games are similar. This text, however, concentrates only on the more complex, four-wall game.

The dimensions and markings on the court are as shown in Figure 1.1. You can easily learn the terminology used to describe the court, floor, ceiling, and front, back, and side walls. The floor lines identify the **service** zone (bounded by the service line and the short line), two rectangular areas called **service boxes**, and the drive serve lines. The only other mark on the court denotes the **receiving line** for the player returning the serve. The floor surface also is divided into playing areas to define court positioning, as shown in Figure 1.2.

Racquetball was invented by Joe Sobek. Using a handball court, he combined the games of handball and squash into a paddle ball game, first called *paddle rackets*, that eventually evolved into today's game of racquetball. The game increased in

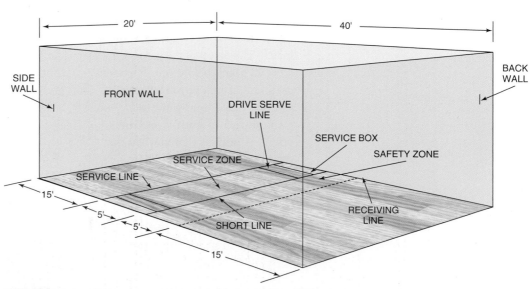

FIGURE 1.1 Dimensions and markings on a racquetball court.

1

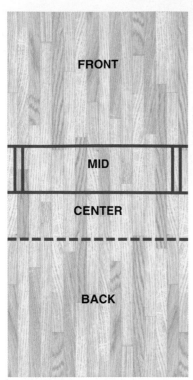

FIGURE 1.2 Designated floor areas on the court.

popularity in the 1970s, and by the late 1970s and early 1980s it had become one of the fastest growing sports in America.

At a point in the mid-1980s, racquetball declined in popularity, but by the late 1980s the decline had leveled off.

Through the 1990s there was a second decline, but by 2001 participation of American players stabilized at 5,296,000, an increase of 2.7 percent from the previous year. The demographics of racquetball have fluctuated over the past 30 years. In 2001 the Sporting Goods Manufacturing Association reported that 25 percent of all participating players were classifed as "frequent player[s]"; of the group, 65.7 percent were male and 34.3 percent female. The 18–34 age group represents the majority of players.

Further, the annual income of American racquetball players is slightly above $69,000, and 51 percent have attended college. Racquetball now is played in more than 90 countries. World championships and the Pan American Games reflect the interest and extent of participation throughout the world.

Overview of the Game

Racquetball is played as a best-of-three match. The object of the game is to score 15 points before your opponent does, and, if each of you wins one game, to play a third game to 11 points.

Only the serving player scores points. A point is scored when the server's opponent fails to hit the ball to the front wall before the ball touches the floor twice. If the server fails to return the ball to the front wall, the server loses serve. In this way, service (and the opportunity to score) alternates until one player or team accumulates 15 points (11 points in the third game) and wins the game.

Racquetball may be played with two (singles), three (cutthroat), or four (doubles) players. In singles, one player opposes another player. In doubles, one two-person team plays another two-person team. In **cutthroat**, a single server plays against two opponents. When the server loses serve, one of the opponents becomes the server and plays against the remaining two players. Scoring is the same as in singles.

In all games, each **rally** (exchange of hits between opposing players) begins with a **legal serve**. For the serve to be legal, the server must stand in the service zone, drop the ball to the floor, and strike it on the rebound so it hits the front wall before any other court surface. The receiver stands between the back of the safety zone line and the back wall in order to return the serve.

To return the serve legally, the receiver must wait until the served ball passes the short line and either bounces in or crosses the safety zone. The front wall rebound may not touch the floor in front of or on the short line. Before the ball hits the floor, it may rebound off one side wall but not off the ceiling, back wall, or both side walls. In the return of serve and any other hit, however, the ball may rebound off any surface except the floor before reaching the front wall.

Service changes when the server fails to keep the ball in play or does not serve legally. If the receiver fails to return the ball to the front wall, the server scores a point.

Outfitting for Play
Clothing

The usual dress for men and women alike is a sports shirt or T-shirt and shorts. Headbands and wristbands are optional (see Photo 1.1A and 1.1B) but aid in absorbing perspiration around the head and hands.

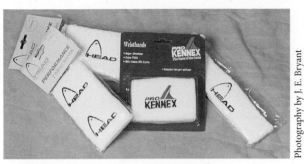

PHOTO 1.1A Racquetball headbands.

Photography by J. E. Bryant

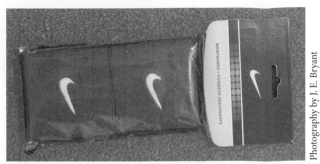

PHOTO 1.1B Racquetball wristbands.

Photography by J. E. Bryant

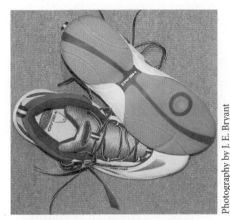

PHOTO 1.2 Racquetball court shoes.

Photography by J. E. Bryant

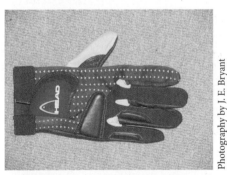

PHOTO 1.3 Racquetball gloves.

Photography by J. E. Bryant

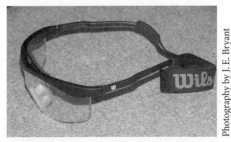

PHOTO 1.4 Protective eyewear.

Photography by J. E. Bryant

Shirts help to absorb body perspiration and must be worn at all times during play. Body perspiration dripping onto the floor of the court presents a potential hazard to cutting and turning associated with footwork.

Shoes

The footwear worn on a racquetball court should be an athletic shoe that supports shifting body weight and lateral movement on the court. Racquetball court shoes (see Photo 1.2) are made specifically for players who take the game seriously. A player can wear tennis shoes or basketball shoes, but they are secondary alternatives to the court shoe.

Shoes designed for running should never be used, and dark-soled shoes also are restricted because they mar court surfaces. Technology has produced an ultra-lightweight court shoe that is designed as a 3/4-top or low-cut shoe.

A court shoe should have excellent traction, comfort, and support. Shoes also should have a full-length midsole for proper cushioning, ventilation, lateral support, and moisture management for breathability and fast drying. Proper footwear also means wearing athletic socks with your court shoes to prevent your feet from sliding in the shoes and creating blisters.

Gloves

Although the use of a glove is optional, players wear a glove on their racquet hand to help maintain better grip on the racquet and prevent the racquet from slipping from their hand. Quality gloves dry soft after use and provide a firm grip to the racquet along with moisture management.

High-performance gloves are made of ultra-thin graphite, Kevlar, and neoprene materials. These materials provide glove strength and durability, as well as padded protection for the knuckles from wall and floor impact. You should look for gloves that provide ventilation and good "feel" to the grip (see Photo 1.3).

Protective Eyewear

Players must wear protective eyewear designed specifically for racquetball players. Competitive rules require pretested eye guards that meet specific safety standards provided by the United States Racquetball Association (USRA) through a list of approved eyewear from companies including Ektelon, ITECH, Leershot, Black Knight, Eagle Eyewear, and Leader. These competitive rules extend to the reputable management of any court facility.

Lensed eyewear is available for players who wear corrective lenses and players who do not wear glasses. Severe eye damage, including detached retinas and the loss of vision, have followed direct eye hits with either the ball or the racquet, and proper protective eyewear dramatically reduces the possibility of eye injury (see Photo 1.4).

The lens must be distortion-free and provide peripheral vision. Lenses are made of polycarbonate material and must be treated with anti-fog and hard-coat treatment that resists scratching.

Players often discard glasses because of fogging. To avoid fogging, the fit of the frame requires a quarter-inch space between the eyebrow and upper rim of the frame. This allows body-generated steam to dissipate without fogging the lens. The frame must be shock-resistant, with soft rubber molded nose pads and temples for comfort and impact protection.

Ball

Specifications for a racquetball ball are determined by the United States Racquetball Association. Although balls come in several colors, most are blue (see Photo 1.5A and B). They are 2 1/4 inches in diameter and weigh 1.6 ounces. When dropped from a 100-inch height at a temperature of 70–74 degrees, the ball should rebound 68 to 72 inches. If it doesn't, it should be replaced with a new ball.

Racquets

Selection of a racquet is dependent upon the style of play, skill level, and amount of money you want to invest. Previously, the frame of the racquet was constructed of materials including aluminum, graphite, fiberglass, and boran. Most racquets today are made of graphite, high-modulus graphite, ultra-high-modulus graphite, Hype Carbon, Tri-Carbon, and titanium (see Photo 1.6). These advanced technologies result in racquets with reduced vibration and greater control, and they generate tremendous power, all of which enhance play.

Racquet sizes and shapes also have changed dramatically. Racquets are now produced from midsize to macro oversize. These sizes extend up to 107 square inches of racquet face and presently are designed in teardrop or quadriform shapes. Racquets are designed to weigh as little as 5 1/2 to 7 ounces, because the larger the hitting surface, the greater the need for the weight of the racquet to be light to maintain maneuverability.

All racquets have a large "sweet spot" that usually is elongated and covers a larger width than the original conventional racquets. Racquet length now can be measured up to 22 inches.

Racquet faces now have longer *mainstrings*, which translate to more power. Larger racquet faces have longer strings, and the longer the string, the more it can stretch. Consequently, the trampoline effect is greater, and thus the power is greater. The more advanced requests are built

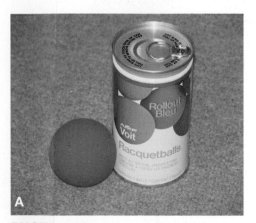

PHOTO 1.5A   Racquetball balls.

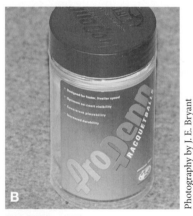

Photography by J. E. Bryant

PHOTO 1.5B   Racquetball balls.

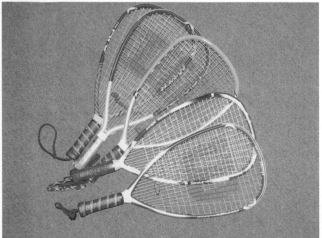

Photography by J. E. Bryant

PHOTO 1.6   22–inch-length racquets.

with a suspended string bed technology that provides increased stability while minimizing shock. It is also important that a racquet weigh 155–195 grams. For the average player, a weight of 155–175 grams is appropriate. Racquets are designed to be balanced head-heavy or head-light. Balance is an individual choice based on feel, but lighter racquets tend to decrease arm injuries. Racquets are strung with various gauges of string: A thin gauge of 17 or 18 provides more power; a heavier gauge of 15 provides a little less power but more durability.

There are accessories for racquets (see Photos 1.7A–D). As examples, tape can be affixed to the racquet to protect the bumper guards and strings from damage caused by striking the walls, and dampening vibrators can be woven through the strings of a racquet to reduce racquet vibration.

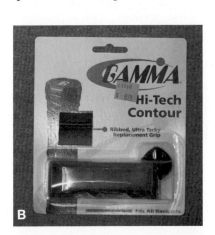

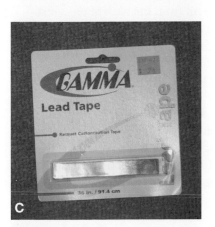

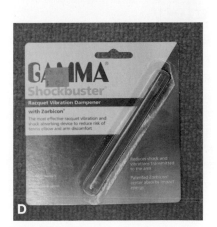

PHOTO 1.7A–D Accessories for racquets and grips.

Photography by J. E. Bryant

Grips and Grip Size

As a rule of thumb, the grip size should be smaller than that of a tennis racquet. Grip sizes range from super-small to medium. Most experts suggest that when gripping the racquet properly, the middle finger of the racquet hand should just touch the palm at the base of the thumb, to allow for a good wrist snap and racquet control.

Racquet Strings and Tension

Often, racquets are already strung when you buy them. When a racquet is strung or restrung, you have to specify the amount of tension. Tension levels are recommended in information accompanying a new racquet, but if you select a tension level on your own, it should range from about 28 to 33 pounds. On the average, players opt for a tension level of approximately 30 ± 4 pounds. The less the string tension, the more power a player has, and the tighter the racquet is strung, the more control. The material used to string is usually monofilament nylon.

Handle and Tether

Racquet handle grips are made of rubber or leather. Although leather is more expensive if tack-treated, it usually allows you to grip the racquet more securely. When selecting a racquet, look for a handle that dampens vibration and reduces wrist fatigue.

The racquet grip has an accessory designed for players who use gloves and players who don't use gloves. These "grippers" provide for a firm grip that enhances the stroke and also serves as a safety feature.

To be legal, each racquet must have a **tether** attached to the handle. The tether is a safety cord worn on the wrist during play. Replacement

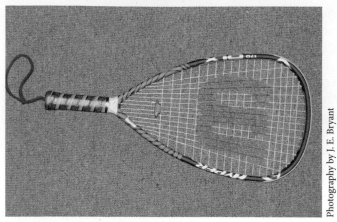

PHOTO 1.8   Safety tether.

Photography by J. E. Bryant

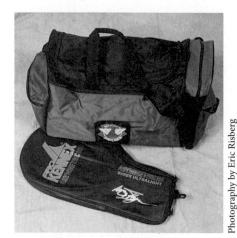

PHOTO 1.9   Bag and cover for racquet.

Photography by Eric Risberg

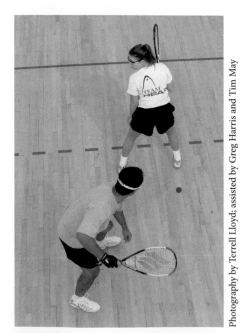

PHOTO 1.10   Hitting a ball when your opponent is in the way.

Photography by Terrell Lloyd; assisted by Greg Harris and Tim May

tethers (see Photo 1.8) may be purchased at stores that sell racquetball equipment.

Racquets are easy to care for if you use some common sense. You should not leave your racquet in the backseat of your car, as extremes in heat or cold will cause the strings to become brittle or break down faster. If you keep a cover on the racquet, it will prevent objects from catching in the strings (see Photo 1.9).

If the strings are breaking frequently, you might insert plastic eyelets where the string wraps around the frame to protect the strings from wearing on the edge and possibly prevent breaking. And be sure to string your racquet with a durable 15-gauge string.

Safety
Safety During Play

Safety on the court begins when you walk onto the court, put on your protective eyewear, and shut the door to prevent people from walking in during play. During play, a racquetball court is safe only if all the players are courteous. This means staying out of your opponent's path to the ball or arm swing. Similarly, no shot is *too good to pass up* if a player is in the path of your swing. There is no

excuse for hitting another player with your racquet. If a player is so close to you that there is a risk of contact, you should stop play rather than continuing (see Photo 1.10).

In addition, you must learn to play the strokes correctly. Too many players keep their tennis stroke alive in the racquetball court. Wide swings from the shoulder require the room a tennis court provides, and there is no place on the racquetball court for this kind of play.

Each racquet must have a tether or safety cord attached to it. This tether is worn around the wrist of the racquet hand to prevent the racquet from flying out of the player's hand and injuring someone on the court. The cord must be used at all times.

Positioning on the court when receiving serve is important. The receiver must remember to wait for the ball to bounce or pass beyond the receiving line of the safety zone before stepping into the zone to return the serve. By doing this, the server is protected from potential serious injury from being hit by the receiver's racquet either at contact with the ball or in the receiver's follow-through.

During play you should continually be aware of players' movements on the court. You must stay out of the way of the player hitting the ball, and when it is your turn to hit, take your shot only if it is clear. Most balls are hit from the back of the court forward. If you are in front of the ball, *do not* turn around completely to "see" what is going on behind you in the back court. This exposes your chest and abdomen to a hard-hit ball and also leaves your face unprotected. Rather, you should angle your body slightly so you can see the back court with your peripheral vision and hold the racquet to protect your face as you look through the strings.

Using the racquet to protect your face from an oncoming ball

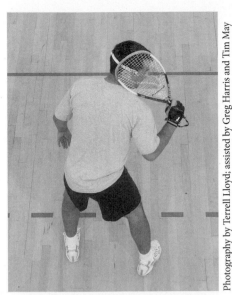

PHOTO 1.11 Protecting your face by looking through the racquet strings.

Photography by Terrell Lloyd; assisted by Greg Harris and Tim May

(see Photo 1.11) is an effective safety measure only if the racquet "beats" the ball to the target. You can't rely on your reflexes to get the racquet up in time to protect your face. As a precaution, you can use your racquet as a shield if your face is exposed to the ball's path, and you must always wear your protective eyewear to protect your eyes against a stray shot. This way, you can play the game and finish still looking the same as when you entered the court.

Experienced players let the ball rebound off the back wall before playing it. This means that a center court position has to be held open for that player to follow the ball. If you anticipate the most direct path to the ball that your opponent can take, you can keep that court position clear. Racquetball is not a game that allows mental lapses. Each player must know where the ball is at all times, and where the other player is moving.

From a safety standpoint, court awareness is related to avoiding interference with your opponent's shot attempt. The term **hinder** is defined as interference with an opponent's shot. Rules regarding hinders are discussed extensively in Chapter 11 under "Hinders." If you interfere with your opponent's movement on the court or with completion of that player's swing, or get hit by your opponent's racquet, a hinder must be called. A hinder should be called by the offended player in a recreational game and by a referee during tournament play.

When a **replay hinder** is called, play is stopped and the point is replayed from the serve. When a penalty hinder is called, play is also stopped, but in this case a loss of rally by the offending player occurs. Contact does not have to occur for a hinder to be requested. Preferably, play should stop before players or racquets collide, to avoid potential injury.

Safety is a matter of habit and thinking. Protect yourself by wearing protective eyewear, using your racquet as a shield, keeping your tether on your wrist, and closing the door of the court when playing. Anticipate your opponent's position, the path of the ball, and the movement of players on the court. Most importantly, remember that racquetball is just a game and one point is not worth risking your well-being or that of your opponent just to make a shot.

Racquetball Injuries

Specific injuries are related to racquetball. A beginning player's injuries tend to be bruises caused by being struck by the ball or by an opponent's racquet, eye injuries from being struck by the ball, sprained ankles, pulled muscles, tendonitis, and blisters on the hands and feet. Most of the injuries result from playing in a small, confined space with another person who has a racquet in his or her hand.

The predictability or unpredictability of an opponent's movement, along with the inexperience of a player, further creates the potential for injury. In addition, the game is designed for strenuous effort, and many individuals attempt to play without proper warm-up or adequate conditioning, which compounds the possibility of injury.

Bruises are part of the game, and as long as a hematoma (severe bruising) does not develop, they are considered minor injuries. Wearing protective clothing, such as sweatpants and top, provides some protection from the potential of bruising caused by being struck by the ball. Having court awareness helps to avoid being hit by an opponent's racquet. Once a bruise, if minor, has formed, treatment usually consists of cold compresses or ice packs to reduce swelling and encourage faster healing.

Eye injuries can be serious. Following preventive safety measures (discussed earlier) is crucial in avoiding this type of injury. The potential for internal damage to the eye, or a detached retina, is significant enough to encourage you to wear protective eyewear. When an eye injury is sustained, medical treatment must be immediate.

Sprained ankles usually are caused by a player making a quick turn without the foot following in the turn, or by lacking awareness of the opponent's position, creating an unexpected foot movement. Muscle strains or pulls result from the same overextension, as well as improper warm-up. As with bruises, initial use of ice or cold compresses can reduce swelling of a sprained ankle or a strain or muscle pull, speeding recovery.

A major caution regarding these types of injuries: Make sure you consult with a medical professional to determine if you have suffered only a minor sprain rather than ligament or tendon damage or a broken bone, as more severe injuries obviously require a totally different treatment.

Tendonitis affecting the elbow usually is caused by too much vibration in the racquet at contact with the ball, too heavy of a racquet, too many hours of play without rest, or incorrect mechanics when executing a backhand stroke. Tendonitis also is found in the shoulder area. This usually is caused by incorrect stroke mechanics or extensive playing time without rest. Characterized by inflammation of the elbow or shoulder joint, these injuries require rest to heal. In some instances, an elbow support or splint can be used as a preventive measure for elbow tendonitis, but nothing replaces proper stroke mechanics in avoiding this type of injury.

Achilles tendon injuries also occur in racquetball. Jumping and landing on the ball of the foot without lowering the heel, or pushing off

the ball of the foot, placing extreme pressure on the tendon, can cause it to rupture. The tendon rupturing sounds like a gunshot report, and the player becomes immediately immobile.

Players often ignore chronic soreness of the Achilles tendon and continue to play. The Achilles tendon and the sheath that surrounds it become inflamed, and soreness, swelling, and pain result. Ignoring these signs can cause severe problems. The only way to address the injury is to stop playing and to rest.

Prevention includes aerobic movement by jogging or use of a treadmill or exercise bike to increase heart rate and blood flow, and by stretching as part of warm-up and warm-down. An orthotic for your shoe is another preventive measure, but elevating your heel also shortens the tendon, when what is needed is to lengthen the tendon. As a result, stretching becomes even more important as a preventive measure. A stiff or achy Achilles tendon is a sign of impending rupture. Rest and consultation with a sports medicine professional are recommended to address the problem.

Blisters are common in most sport participation situations but usually can be avoided in racquetball. Blisters are caused by moisture, pressure, or friction. Hand blisters are caused by an improper grip size and extensive play that causes a "hot spot" on the hand. This type of blister can be avoided by using the proper racquet grip size and by wearing a racquetball glove during play.

Blisters that develop on the feet usually are caused by friction from feet sliding in the shoe. To address this situation, wear a pair of cotton socks with insoles as a preventive measure. Using appropriate shoes designed for court play that manages moisture can also go a long way in preventing blisters. Once blisters have developed, the main concern is to make sure they do not get infected. For a foot blister, an athletic trainer can create a doughnut-shaped pad to reduce the pain at the pressure point and thereby allow you to continue to play.

Racquetball requires quick turns, stops, and starts. Repetitive twisting and trunk rotation are a part of racquetball. The risk of back injury increases because of the movement required in the game. Preventive measures include a total conditioning program, proper stretching (see Chapter 2), and sound stroke technique.

From an injury standpoint, there is also the danger of dehydration as well as cramps, which can make participation in racquetball uncomfortable. Older racquetball courts often do not have good air circulation; consequently, the environment can become very warm. Intake of liquids will assist in avoiding cramps and dehydration. (Chapter 2 provides further information on fluid intake.)

If you follow safety procedures, your racquetball experience will be relatively injury-free and also more enjoyable. If an injury does occur, immediate attention to the injury will hasten recovery.

Resources

Many racquetball resources are available for your use. The United States Racquetball Association (USRA) provides the official rules and publishes a magazine four times per year, entitled *Racquetball Magazine*, for its members along with a newsletter eight times per year. In addition, the USRA produces instructional materials including DVDs entitled *Beginning Racquetball* and *Secrets of the Pros* by Jim Winterton and a video, *Building Your Racquetball Dream House*, by Fran Davis. The USRA sanctions age-group and various skill-level tournaments,

sponsors regional associations, trains and certifies players and instructors, and generally promotes racquetball at the grassroots level. One of its noteworthy efforts is the promotion of racquetball for disabled athletes, including those who use a wheelchair and individuals who have visual and hearing impairments. The USRA offers a membership that includes a subscription to *Racquetball Magazine*.*

Resources also include professional instruction and coaching. Nearly every college and university offers racquetball as a course for students. In addition, fitness and sports clubs usually have an instructor available for lessons, along with a series of racquetball functions including local tournaments for all ages and skill levels. When taking racquetball lessons, questions you should ask of an instructor include:

- How much individual time will you provide me? (The more individual time, the better.)
- What will you teach me? (You need to develop as a player rather than repeat past learning experiences.)
- What kind of teaching credentials do you have? (Anyone can attempt to teach racquetball, but USRA instructor status or a teaching credential associated with racquetball is critical.)

Countless equipment manufacturers support racquetball, contributing to your racquetball development. Ektelon is a good example of a corporation that produces excellent equipment and also provides instructional materials on how to play racquetball. Its website is http://www.ektelon.com. Other companies, including Wilson, E-Force, and Head, also support

---

* The USRA requires a $25 membership fee for college students. The membership application address is: USRA, 1685 West Uintah, Colorado Springs, CO 80904-2906, or www.usra.org, or call 719/635-5396.

development of the game. The Internet provides many additional resources. To order instructional videotapes on racquetball, you can access http://www.masterball.com and find two videotapes: *Mastery of Racquetball—Doubles*, and *Mastery of Racquetball—The Complete Success Program* (*Singles*). There are countless other racquetball websites, most of which provide information on equipment or instruction, which you can access by simply entering the key word *racquetball*.

POINTS *to* REMEMBER

Do put on your protective eyewear before entering the court.

Do shut the door to the court before you begin hitting.

Do keep the tether of the racquet securely on your wrist.

Do know where the ball is at all times.

Do remember that winning a point is never worth injuring an opponent.

Don't swing at the ball if your opponent is in the way.

Don't turn around completely to see what is going on behind you.

CHECKPOINTS

Answers are located on page 141.

1. A legal match score is:
   a. 15–13, 7–15, 15–10
   b. 21–17, 21–3
   c. 13–15, 15–6, 11–10
   d. 13–15, 15–13, 15–14

2. A legal serve consists of the following:
   a. Server stands in the service zone. After the server bounces the ball and strikes it, the ball must hit the front wall first and then clear the short line and bounce before striking a second wall.
   b. Server stands in the service zone. After the server bounces the ball and strikes it, the ball must hit the front wall first and then clear the short line, striking no more than one side wall before bouncing on the floor.
   c. Server stands in the service zone. After the server bounces the ball and strikes it, the ball must hit the front wall first and then clear the short line before striking the back wall.
   d. Server stands in the service zone. After the server bounces the ball

and strikes it, the ball may hit one side wall before hitting the front wall first and then clear the short line before striking the floor.

3. The receiver of serve may return the serve by:
   a. contacting the ball and striking a side wall and front wall, followed by the ball making contact with the floor.
   b. contacting the ball and striking the ceiling and front wall, followed by the ball making contact with the floor.
   c. contacting the ball and striking the front wall, followed by the ball making contact with the floor.
   d. all of the above.

4. When the ball has been placed into play, it may be:
   a. hit on the fly.
   b. hit after it bounces once.
   c. hit after two bounces.
   d. both a and b.

5. Shirts must be worn because they:
   a. look good.
   b. absorb sweat.

   c. provide the opponent with visual contact.
   d. all of the above.

6. Characteristics of quality protective eyewear include:
   a. polycarbonate material.
   b. non-scratch lenses.
   c. non-fog lenses.
   d. all of the above.

7. The modern racquetball racquets length must be no longer than:
   a. 21 inches.
   b. 22 inches.
   c. 23 inches.
   d. 24 inches.

8. The lone safety rule that is not a specific game rule is:
   a. Tether cord must be attached to wrist when ball is in play.
   b. Racquet must be held in front of face when ball is being played behind player.
   c. Player must wear protective eyewear.
   d. Server must not hit serve before ball has bounced or passed beyond the receiving line of safety zone.

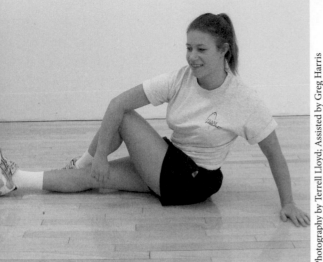

Photography by Terrell Lloyd; Assisted by Greg Harris and Tim May

2

Preparation for Play

To use their skills and strategy to the best advantage, racquetball players must maintain proper physical conditioning. With less-than-optimal fitness, fatigue sets in too quickly, injuries are more likely to occur, and the quality of play declines. Although the optimal level of fitness for each player is an individual decision based upon the quality of play he or she wants to maintain, conditioning for all levels of play has to be a year-round activity.

Physical conditioning is not like learning to ride a bicycle (once you have it, you never lose it). Instead, the state of conditioning is transient and responds to the amount of use or disuse of the body. If the body is not "used" in exercise, it loses strength and endurance. This is not to imply that physical conditioning will improve your racquetball skills. If you want to be a better racquetball player, you must play racquetball. Optimal conditioning, however, will allow you to get the best out of your skills.

Some components of physical conditioning should be trained weekly regardless of whether you are playing racquetball. Thus, when play begins, you are ready to play your best. Most people make the mistake of trying to condition for a sport at the same time they are starting to play. This increase in activity overloads the body and it "breaks down." Either an actual injury occurs or general fatigue takes away the pleasure of the game. Ideally, the racquetball player should always be "fit" to play. Minimally, to be fit means that you have conditioned your body aerobically and with weight training.

Aerobic Conditioning for Recovery

Although success in racquetball relies on quickness, skill, and strategy, none of these factors will be important if you are too tired to move. During rallies, most of the energy the body uses is a product of **anaerobic metabolism**, the release of energy without the use of oxygen. Restoring these energy supplies for the next rally, however, requires oxygen. Therefore, although energy needs during play are not primarily **aerobic** ("with oxygen"), the more oxygen that can be inhaled between rallies, the faster you can recover and the less tired you will become during the game. This means that part of your physical conditioning program must involve **aerobic conditioning**—training to bring oxygen into the body, circulate it to the muscles, and utilize it efficiently to recover quickly.

Before beginning any aerobic conditioning program, you should make sure it is safe for your body. As a general rule, if you are under 35, have had a thorough physical in the last year, and have no reason to suspect you are less than healthy, you can begin exercising immediately. If you have not had a medical checkup in a year or more, suspect that you might have hypertension or diabetes, are extremely overweight (more than 20 percent over your suggested weight), use tobacco products, or have other health problems (such as back problems), you should check with your physician before starting an aerobic conditioning program.

If you are over 35, you should have medical clearance from your physician. Make sure your physician understands the type of program in which you want to get involved. If you obtain clearance, you are ready to begin.

Among the variety of activities to train your body aerobically are walking, running, cross-country skiing, swimming, and bicycling, as well as aerobic exercise classes (dance, bench stepping, and so on). These activities are good conditioners because they require an increase in oxygen to be brought into the body during the activity. This allows your system to literally "practice" oxygen utilization.

Although any of these activities may be used, a jog–run program is suggested because racquetball requires you to run around the court. Just going out for a brisk walk may or may not be helpful in improving your conditioning for this sport because this activity may not stress your body adequately. For aerobic conditioning to occur, certain guidelines must be followed. These guidelines define how hard you must exercise (intensity), how long (duration), and how often (frequency)

for the exercise to be safe, yet difficult enough for training to result.

Intensity

In general, the intensity of exercise is monitored by your heart rate. For most people under age 35, exercising between 70 percent and 85 percent of the maximal heart rate will provide adequate intensity. **Maximal heart rate** is the maximal speed your heart can beat when exercising as hard as you can.

One way to predict your maximal heart rate is to subtract your age from 220. For an individual under 35, to calculate the proper exercise intensity, determine 70 percent and 85 percent of this number. This formula gives the exercise heart rate range.

For example, a man who is 28 years old would have a predicted maximal heart rate of 192 (220 minus 28). His exercise heart rate range would be 134 (70 percent) to 163 (85 percent) beats per minute. Ideally, to train aerobically, your heart must be beating at a speed within this range.

For individuals between 35 and 50 years of age, the range is slightly different. Exercising between 60 percent and 70 percent of your maximal heart rate identifies an appropriate level of activity. Because activity levels in this group are so variable, you can work at a higher intensity after several exercise sessions if you are in good aerobic condition and the lower intensity seems too easy.

To make sure you are not exercising above your capabilities, use the "talk test" as a guide. During aerobic conditioning you should be able to talk and exercise at the same time. If you cannot, you are working too hard and are not bringing in enough oxygen to match the exercise intensity. This means *slow down*. If you find that 60 percent to 70 percent is too hard, lower your intensity. As conditioning progresses, you will be able to move into the higher exercise heart rate range. Give yourself time to condition for it.

Finally, individuals 50 and older should begin at an intensity between 50 percent and 60 percent of their predicted maximal heart rate. Again, use the talk test as your guide, and regulate your exercise accordingly.

To check your heart rate, exercise for at least 5 minutes, then stop and take a 10-second count of your heartbeat. Use the pulse in your neck at the carotid artery, or the pulse at your wrist. Count the first beat you feel in the 10-second count as 0. At the end of the time period, multiply the number of beats counted by 6 to determine if the number of beats per minute falls within the exercise heart rate range. If it is above the range, slow down. If it is below, speed up, unless the talk test suggests otherwise.

Duration

Now that you are working at the proper intensity, how long must you exercise at this level? Anywhere between 15 and 60 minutes will provide enough time to give your body sufficient practice at using oxygen. In general, 20 to 30 minutes is recommended as the proper exercise duration. This means 20 to 30 minutes of constant, nonstop exercise at your exercise heart rate.

If this level of activity is too difficult for you to begin with, start with a jog–walk interval program. Begin by jogging a few minutes, and then walk until you are ready to jog again. Keep track of the time you spent jogging versus walking.

Each week, try to increase the amount of time jogging and decrease the walking time until you can jog the entire 20 minutes. Don't be afraid to jog slowly. This is a conditioning activity, not a race!

Frequency

How often should you do aerobic conditioning? Three to four times a week is ideal, and five times is tolerated well. Participating in more than five aerobic exercise sessions a week could result in an increased rate of injuries to muscles and joints.

For the exercise sessions to be of most value, give yourself between 24 and 48 hours of rest between each aerobic workout. The more out of shape you are, the more recovery time you will need. If your recovery time is longer than 48 hours, some detraining in aerobic conditioning will occur. Therefore, you should keep your program regular in frequency but sensible in stress to balance your exercise needs with your capabilities.

Aerobic conditioning should be a basis for all your sports programs and, as such, should be done consistently throughout the year. When you are playing more racquetball, however, you may find that you have to cut back on aerobic conditioning because of time constraints or energy limitations. Cutting back to two exercise sessions a week will just maintain aerobic conditioning without developing it.

Therefore, if you must decrease your aerobic exercise, maintain at least two aerobic sessions a week to completely avoid detraining in this capacity. Your heart won't get any stronger, but at least you should minimize deconditioning. Developing your physical condition takes time and effort, but you have the rest of your life to work at it.

Weight Training: Developing Strength and Endurance

Muscular strength and **endurance** help provide power to your racquetball stroke. Without adequate "muscle" behind each shot, the speed of the ball will be compromised. Muscular endurance helps to maintain this power during long rallies or throughout a prolonged match. These two muscle capabilities go hand in hand and should be developed simultaneously to get the most benefit for play.

One of the best ways to develop strength and endurance is through weight training. For racquetball, this training should be concentrated on the muscles of the arms, shoulders, chest, upper back, abdominals, and legs. How do you know if you have adequate strength in these muscles?

1. Do you fail to hit the ball consistently as hard as you want, given that you are using the proper technique?

2. Do your legs get tired, especially after a long rally?

If your answer to either question is "yes," weight training may be helpful in improving the quality of your game. Before beginning a weight training program, follow the same precautions given for aerobic conditioning, and check with your physician to determine if this is a safe activity for you.

To improve strength and endurance, weight training should be done two or three times a week (preferably on the days you are not training aerobically). Ideally, when you are not playing racquetball weekly, you should concentrate on improving your strength through these two or three workouts per week. During your racquetball season, you can maintain strength with one hard workout a week. Unlike aerobic conditioning, strength gains are retained for a longer time and don't require exercise as often to prevent detraining.

The question, then, is which weight training exercises will be most helpful for playing racquetball? The following are some exercises that are beneficial for strengthening the muscles needed to play.

Chest Press

Abdominal Crunch

Leg Press

Upright Rowing

Bent-arm Pullover

Leg Curl

Shoulder Press

Wrist Curls

Leg Extension

Triceps Extension

Each exercise should be done with 8 to 10 repetitions for 3 sets. Begin by using a weight that fatigues you to exhaustion in the third set. When you can complete this number of lifts comfortably, you can either increase the weight lifted (to increase strength) or increase the number of repetitions per set (to increase endurance).

Beginning weight training books, which include lifting techniques and safety concerns, are available at your local college bookstore. Books used by a college weight training class typically give excellent hints about weight training effectively and safely. If you still have questions, ask the supervisor in a weight training room at a college or fitness center.

If you do not have access to a weight training room, calisthenics can be utilized to increase muscular strength and endurance. Exercises such as push-ups, crunches, and chin-ups, done in sets similar to weight training, will provide a stimulus for strengthening. You can begin with 5 sets of 10 repetitions each. Rest 30 to 60 seconds between sets. If this level of exercise is too easy, increase the number of repetitions per set, rather than the number of sets, until you find a challenging routine.

Stair-climbing or bench-stepping can be beneficial in developing leg strength. If you are running up a stairway, give yourself three times as long to recover as it took to run the stairs. For example, if you completed the stairs in 10 seconds, wait 30 seconds before repeating the climb. Repeat the stairs as many times as your condition allows.

When stepping on a bench, step up and down with 1 leg, repeating the movement 10 to 15 times, then switch legs. You may or may not need to rest when switching legs, depending on your condition. Try to complete five sets with each leg.

Improvement in strength and endurance takes time, but if you stay with it, your racquetball game will improve simply because you are in better condition to play. However, just being in good condition will not help if you do not prepare yourself physically and mentally to play before you enter the court. It is just as important to warm up your "engine" before a racquetball game as it is to keep yourself in good condition.

The Warm-up

Whenever you are beginning to exercise, a rule of thumb is this: Never take your body by surprise. A **warm-up** to prepare yourself mentally and physically allows your body to shift gears smoothly from inactivity to activity. Without a warm-up, the stress of sudden activity can cause your body to rely on reserve energy sources normally used only during emergencies. Using your reserve

energy at the start of the exercise can cause you to fatigue more quickly and adversely affect your level of play.

The warm-up consists of three phases: *relaxation*, *increased heart activity*, and *stretching*.

Relaxation

Relaxation is needed to relieve internal stress. The body responds to stress by increasing muscle tension. Tight muscles work in opposition to the free and fluid movement needed for any exercise or sport activity. In addition, any stretching exercises you do will be more effective if the muscles are relaxed first. To relax, sit comfortably with your eyes closed for several minutes. Concentrate only on your breathing, remembering to exhale completely.

Increased Heart Activity

The second phase of the warm-up should increase your heart rate. This activity also will speed the release of the body's available energy. As a result, at the beginning of the game, the reserve energy stores are not utilized. Playing racquetball will feel more comfortable, and you will not tire as rapidly.

Bench-stepping, rope-skipping, and running in place (see Photos 2.1, 2.2, and 2.3) are examples of activities that will increase your heart rate. These activities should be done at low-to-moderate intensity. Your breathing should increase, but not to the point of your being out of breath.

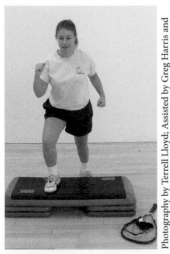

PHOTO 2.1   Bench-stepping.

Photography by Terrell Lloyd; Assisted by Greg Harris and Tim May

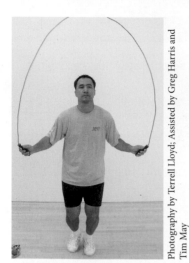

PHOTO 2.2   Rope-skipping.

Photography by Terrell Lloyd; Assisted by Greg Harris and Tim May

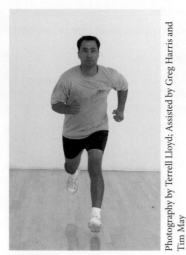

PHOTO 2.3   Running in Place.

Photography by Terrell Lloyd; Assisted by Greg Harris and Tim May

This phase of the warm-up is finished when you begin to "break a sweat," usually in 3–5 minutes.

Stretching

Now that the body is warm, you can begin the last phase of the warm-up, stretching. Stretching is important to increase your ease and range of movement, referred to as **flexibility**. Although racquetball shots ideally should be hit just below waist level, there are opportunities for overhead strokes and returns when you must extend your arm to reach a ball. Flexibility in the shoulder joint will allow these movements to be done comfortably.

In addition, a player needs freedom of movement through the back to twist and turn, and through the hips and legs to bend and squat. If muscles are tight, movement is limited, detracting from your ability to reach the ball in different parts of the court with different strokes. Stretching exercises can ensure that you maintain the maximum range of movement in the joints of your body.

Ideally, stretching exercises are done every day. If you are going to play racquetball, stretching should be included as part of your warm-up before play and cool-down afterward.

Stretching before play helps to loosen the joints and muscles to prepare for fast movements of the body during the game. After play, as you are cooling down, stretching helps to relieve contractions in fatigued muscles and prevent tight muscles the next day.

The stretching exercises presented here by no means comprise an exhaustive list of all exercises that can be done. Your favorites may be missing. Add them if they are helpful to you. The following stretches, however, do involve all major muscles used when playing racquetball. The basis for most of these stretches is extrapolated from Werner W. K. Hoeger's *Lifetime Physical Fitness & Wellness: A Personalized Program* (Belmont, CA: Wadsworth Publishing, 2003).

Whichever exercises you do, you should follow several basic rules. Start with the head and work down the body, stretching the large muscles first and then the small muscles. Never bounce into a stretched position. Trying to "force" a stretch contracts the muscle instead of allowing it to lengthen. Obviously, this is contrary to the purpose of the stretch. To avoid contracting the muscle, hold the stretch position without moving (except to breathe). This static position allows the muscle to relax and lengthen. Once the muscle is relaxed during a stretch, you may want to try to stretch the muscle further to increase your range of motion.

Each static stretch should last at least 15 seconds and be repeated 3 to 5 times. This means that completing the set of stretching exercises will take a minimum of 10–15 minutes. If you choose to go back and repeat some exercises, plan to spend more time working on your flexibility rather than skip other stretches. If you are excessively sore the next morning after playing, stretch your sore muscles periodically throughout the day. Many of the stretches illustrated here can be done in street

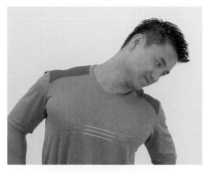
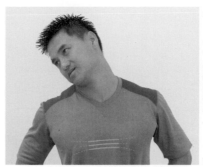

Photography by Terrell Lloyd; Assisted by Greg Harris and Tim May

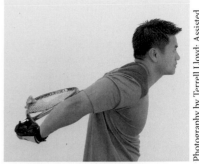

Photography by Terrell Lloyd; Assisted by Greg Harris and Tim May

Lateral Head Tilt

Action: Tilt the head slowly and gently to one side. Pull down with the opposite shoulder. Hold the stretch 15 seconds. Alternate to the other side. Repeat as needed.

Areas stretched: Flexors and extensors, and ligaments of the cervical spine.

Shoulder Hyperextension Stretch

Action: Grasp the throat of racquet with hands close together. Slowly bring the arms up to as close to a perpendicular position to the body as possible. Hold the stretch 15 seconds. Repeat as needed.

Areas stretched: Deltoid and pectoral muscles and ligaments of the shoulder joint.

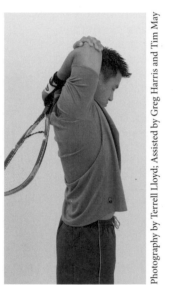

Photography by Terrell Lloyd; Assisted by Greg Harris and Tim May

Shoulder and Arm Stretch

Action: Place the racquet head in the small of the back with the elbow in an *up* position. Place the nonracquet hand above the elbow and apply minimal pressure downward to place the shoulder area on stretch. Hold the stretch 15 seconds. Repeat as needed. (NOTE: You can do this same stretch with your non-racquet arm to relieve tension in this area.)

Areas stretched: Ligaments of the shoulder joint and triceps muscle.

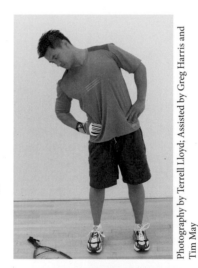

Photography by Terrell Lloyd; Assisted by Greg Harris and Tim May

Side Stretch

Action: Stand with feet spread to shoulder width and hands on hips. Without moving the feet or bending at the knees or hips, lean to one side. Do not bend forward. Hold stretch for 15 seconds. Repeat to the other side. Repeat as needed.

Areas stretched: Intercostal muscles and ligaments of rib cage, muscles and ligaments of pelvis.

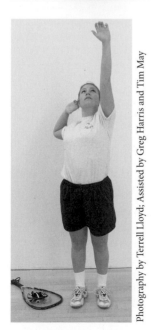

Photography by Terrell Lloyd; Assisted by Greg Harris and Tim May

Ladder Climb

Action: While standing straight and looking up, reach as high as possible with each arm alternately. Hold the stretched position for 15 seconds before changing arms. Repeat as needed.

Areas stretched: Shoulder girdle and upper back muscles.

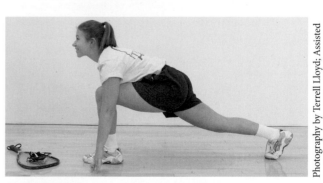

Photography by Terrell Lloyd; Assisted by Greg Harris and Tim May

Groin Stretch

Action: Place one foot between hands, placed on floor, shoulder-width apart. Lean forward with back leg stretched as far as possible. Try to keep forward leg bent at 90-degree angle. Hold 15 seconds. Switch legs. Repeat as needed.

Areas stretched: Groin and hip flexor muscles and ligaments.

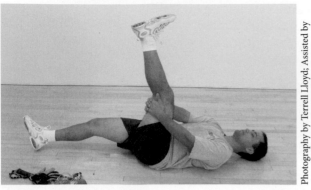

Photography by Terrell Lloyd; Assisted by Greg Harris and Tim May

Hamstring Stretch

Action: Lying on floor with one leg extended and slightly bent, elevate opposite leg straight into the air. With both hands, gently pull on hamstring, bringing the leg closer to the upper body. Hold 15 seconds. Alternate legs, and repeat as needed.

Areas stretched: Lower back and lumbar spine ligaments, hamstring muscle.

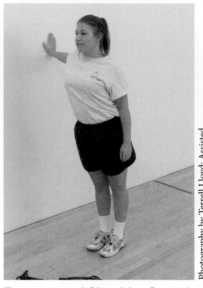

Photography by Terrell Lloyd; Assisted by Greg Harris and Tim May

Forearm and Shoulder Stretch

Action: Stand arm's length away from wall. Place palm of hand on wall at shoulder height. Rotate shoulder forward while keeping hand in place. Hold 15 seconds. Alternate hands. Repeat as needed.

Areas stretched: Deltoid, biceps, forearm flexor muscles, and forearm ligaments.

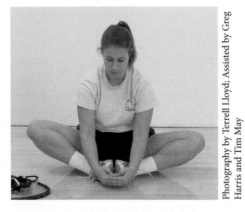

Photography by Terrell Lloyd; Assisted by Greg Harris and Tim May

Butterfly

Action: Sit on floor with soles of your feet touching. Place your feet as close to your body as possible. Pull your trunk toward the floor. Hold 15 seconds. Repeat as needed.

Areas stretched: Lower back and spine, hip adductor muscles.

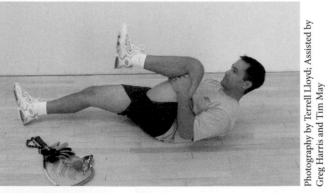

Photography by Terrell Lloyd; Assisted by Greg Harris and Tim May

Single Knee to Chest Stretch

Action: Lie flat on padded surface. Bend one leg and place both hands on the hamstring side of the thigh. Pull this leg toward your chest. Hold 15 seconds. Change legs. Repeat as needed.

Areas stretched: Lower back and hamstring muscles, lumbar spine ligaments.

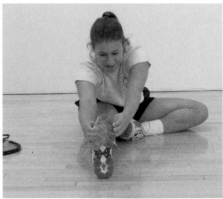

Photography by Terrell Lloyd; Assisted by Greg Harris and Tim May

Modified Hurdler's Stretch

Action: On floor with one leg extended and sole of other foot touching inner thigh, slowly reach as far forward as possible. Pull upper body down. Hold 15 seconds. Repeat as needed.

Areas stretched: Hamstrings and lower back muscles, lumbar spine ligaments.

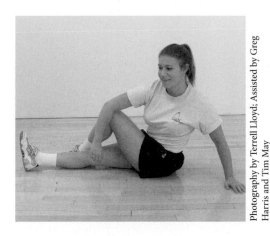

Photography by Terrell Lloyd; Assisted by Greg Harris and Tim May

Trunk Twist

Action: Sit on floor and bend your left leg, placing your left foot on the outside of your right knee. Place your right elbow on your left knee and push against it. At the same time, try to rotate the trunk to the left (counterclockwise). Hold 15 seconds. Change to the other side. Repeat as needed.

Areas stretched: Lateral side of hip and trunk; trunk and lower back.

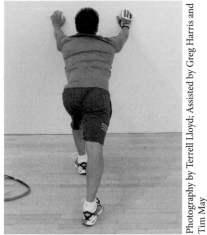

Photography by Terrell Lloyd; Assisted by Greg Harris and Tim May

Heel Cord Stretch

Action: Stand 2–3 feet away from a wall. Stretch heel of the back foot downward. Hold 15 seconds. Alternate feet. Repeat as needed.

Areas stretched: Achilles tendon, gastrocnemius and soleus muscles.

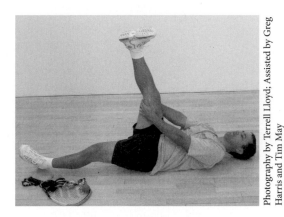

Photography by Terrell Lloyd; Assisted by Greg Harris and Tim May

Ankle Stretch

Action: Using the same position as the Hamstring Stretch, alternately turn toes of elevated foot inward, then outward. Hold each position 15 seconds. When finished, slowly rotate your ankle through these positions. Alternate feet. Repeat as needed.

Areas stretched: Muscles and ligaments of ankle and lower leg.

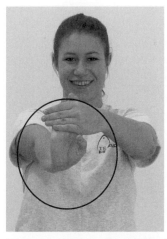 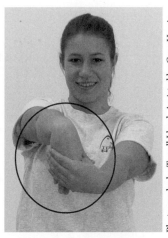

Photography by Terrell Lloyd; Assisted by Greg Harris and Tim May

Wrist and Forearm Stretch

Action: Holding your left hand against your right hand, gently pull back against your fingers. Hold 15 seconds, then push your fingers down. Hold 15 seconds. Reverse hands and stretch. Repeat as needed.

Areas stretched: Forearm flexors and extensor muscles, wrist ligaments.

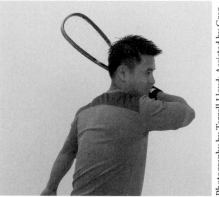

Photography by Terrell Lloyd; Assisted by Greg Harris and Tim May

Serving Motion and Rotation

Action: With your racquet in your hand and your arm extended in front of you, pull your arm through an arc and rotate your body until the racquet is directly behind you. Hold this position. Come forward slowly with the racquet as if stroking a ball, rotating your body forward. Complete the "swing" with a follow-through of the stroke. Turn your body as far as possible to exaggerate the follow-through, and hold this position 15 seconds. Repeat as needed.

Areas stretched: Hip, abdominal, chest, back, neck, and shoulder muscles; hip and spinal ligaments.

clothes, sitting in a chair, or even standing up.

If the more you stretch, the more sore the muscle becomes, STOP! You may be dealing with an injury rather than a tight muscle. Persistent or increasing pain is a signal that you should rest or even see a doctor.

The three warm-up phases should be done in sequence immediately before entering the court to play. Many people make the mistake of warming up and then waiting 5–10 minutes before playing racquetball. Consequently, most of the effect of the warm-up is lost. The increase in heart rate will decline within one to two minutes after the warm-up is over. Therefore, no time should be wasted getting onto the court.

Mental Readiness

Racquetball is played in an enclosed area with at least one other competitor. Too often, the game is played as a power game with the potential for intimidation. Unless your mind is focused on your game and skill execution rather than on your opponent, you will not perform at your best. More important, when in the court, this is a time to forget about your work, ignore outside noises and distractions, and eliminate self-doubt about your play. This is a time to be mentally ready to play. Mental readiness includes being focused on the court, concentrating on shots, and displaying mental toughness during the game.

Focus

The physical warm-up that is done prior to play is intended to prepare your mind and body for your time on the court. This preparation is wasted unless you can focus your thoughts on the game ahead rather than what happened yesterday or where you need to be after you finish play. Remember, you have chosen this game! Enjoy it by focusing your senses—hearing, touch, smell—on the environment you are in, a racquetball court! This will allow you to enjoy the game more and also will help you to play better because you won't be distracted. For the time you are in the court, this is your world!

Concentration

Concentration allows you to execute shots to the best of your ability. If you want to improve your game, you must think about what you are doing on the court. Well-executed shots don't just happen; they are a result of purposeful action. You must concentrate on the action in the game as long as the rally continues.

Don't congratulate yourself on a well-placed shot before the point is over. Think about where to place your next shot and mentally stay in the play until it is completed. Losing your concentration on the court prevents you from playing your best and also can lead to injury if you lose the sense of where your opponent is positioned on the court.

If you are having trouble maintaining concentration, try to relax by taking several deep breaths. Focus on the exhale of each breath and re-center your thoughts to this moment in time, not to what just happened. Give yourself a few encouraging words and constructive advice (for example, "I need to prepare earlier for my 'shot'; I have to keep moving my feet on the court").

Concentrate on what will help you play better, not on your frustrations at your mistakes.

Mental Toughness

Racquetball, especially at the beginner's level, is often played as a power game. Hitting the ball hard, rather than placing the ball accurately, often becomes the immediate goal. As a result, beginning players often are hit with the ball during play. Also, beginning players don't always execute shots correctly. Skill improvement is part of learning!

To play your best, you cannot allow the power of the opponent's shot, the pain of being hit by an errant ball, or your own frustration with your play get in the way of continuing to improve. Hiding in the corner of the court because you are intimidated by your opponent or worrying about whether you will repeat the same mishit will not aid your game. Recognize that you are learning the game, visualize yourself hitting the ball perfectly, and eagerly anticipate your next opportunity to hit a winning shot.

Above all, don't give up! Play every point hard, learn from your mistakes, and don't lose your temper. If your opponent thinks he or she has conquered you mentally, it provides a positive reinforcement for more aggressive play on your opponent's part.

The more you can stay calm during play, focus on the world in the court, and concentrate on your shots and your opponent's play, the more likely you will be to play your best. After all, isn't this your primary goal?

The Need for Fluids

Of special concern to racquetball players is overheating and dehydration. Prolonged **hyperthermia** (elevated body temperature) may lead to heat cramps, heat exhaustion, and heatstroke. Any of these conditions can arise when you are playing in a hot court for an extended time and have lost a lot of body fluid through sweating (see Photo 2.4). Although heat cramps are painful and temporarily disabling, they are not life-threatening. Untreated **heatstroke**, however, can be fatal.

To prevent problems associated with **dehydration** and overheating, make sure your clothing allows for good air circulation around your body. Avoid clothing that traps heat and promotes excessive sweating. This causes you to lose more body fluids.

Body fluids are important in regulating body temperature. If you lose too many fluids, your body is likely to overheat, just like the radiator of your car when its water level is low. Some sweating is necessary to keep the body cool, however. Thus, the key to successful participation in a hot environment is to maintain an adequate level of body fluids by drinking.

To determine how much water to drink, a rule of thumb is, "A pint's a pound the world around." For every pound of weight lost during exercise, you should drink a pint of water. To determine this amount, weigh yourself before and after playing, and drink a pint of water for each pound difference.

If you will be playing racquetball for more than 30 minutes, you should start replacing body fluids even before you begin the activity. Cold water (50° Fahrenheit) is best when taken in small amounts (3 to 6 ounces). Continue to drink 3 to 6 ounces at 10–15 minute intervals during the game.

Because water is what is being lost from the body, water is needed to replace body fluids. For most people, electrolyte replacement solutions (such as Gatorade) are not needed during exercise, although they aid recovery after play is over.

If proper fluid levels are maintained by drinking water before, during, and after playing, overheating should not be a problem. Moreover, you will not fatigue as quickly during the game. For your own safety, begin each game of racquetball with a drink of water!

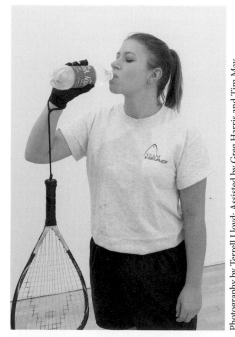

Photography by Terrell Lloyd. Assisted by Greg Harris and Tim May

PHOTO 2.4   Start Each Game with a Drink of Water.

POINTS *to* REMEMBER

Before playing, prepare your body with a good warm-up. The warm-up should relax your body, increase your heart rate, and stretch your muscles.

For your warm-up to be effective, complete the warm-up just before entering the court.

During play, block out extraneous thoughts and concentrate only on each shot; control your temper and learn from your mistakes.

Avoid wearing clothing that traps heat and promotes excessive sweating.

Drink 3–6 ounces of cold water every 10–15 minutes during the match.

After playing, drink a pint of water for every pound of weight lost.

CHECKPOINTS

Answers are located on page 141.

1. The three phases identified with a proper warm-up are:
   a. relaxation, increased heart rate, stretching.
   b. relaxation, decreased heart rate, stretching.
   c. psyching up, increased heart rate, stretching.
   d. psyching up, relaxation, stretching.

2. When stretching:
   a. begin at the head and work down the body.
   b. stretch the small muscles first and then the large muscles.
   c. bounce on stretches.
   d. force a stretch to ensure a good stretch.

3. Stretching assists a player before beginning competition to
   a. relieve muscle contraction and prevent tight muscles.
   b. avoid fatiguing muscles.
   c. loosen the joints and muscles to prepare for fast movements.
   d. all of the above.

4. Mental readiness requires a player to:
   a. be mentally tough.
   b. concentrate on playing the game.
   c. block outside influences.
   d. all of the above.

5. When playing more than 30 minutes during a game, a player should consume:
   a. 3 ounces of liquid every 5–10 minutes.
   b. 3–6 ounces of liquid every 10–15 minutes.
   c. 3–6 ounces of liquid every 15–20 minutes.
   d. 6–9 ounces of liquid every 30 minutes.

6. Which of the following stretches help prepare the upper body for activity?
   a. Hamstring stretch
   b. Ladder climb
   c. Butterfly
   d. Groin stretch

7. To be most effective, a stretch should be:
   a. bounced into and repeated 3–5 times.
   b. done only on the racquet side of the body.
   c. from a static position and held for at least 15 seconds.
   d. avoided if you are sore the next day.

8. If, when stretching, the muscle becomes sore, you should:
   a. stop stretching.
   b. ease off, but keep exercising.
   c. increase effort.
   d. stop for a 30–60 second period and then stretch again.

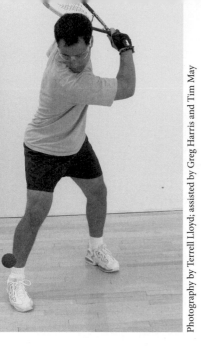

Photography by Terrell Lloyd; assisted by Greg Harris and Tim May

Preliminaries to the Strokes in Racquetball

Being properly prepared to hit the ball is essential to executing offensive and defensive shots correctly. This includes gripping the racquet properly, assuming the set or ready position, and pivoting to either a forehand or a backhand hitting position.

Holding the Racquet: the Grips

The power in a racquetball stroke comes from the snap of the wrist when the ball is contacted. Unless the racquet is gripped in a way that maximizes this snap, the potential power of a stroke will be lost.

Most players use two basic grips during play. A third type of grip may be used in special situations. The first, and easily the most popular, is the Eastern forehand grip. The Eastern forehand grip, as its name implies, is used to hit only shots on the racquet-hand (forehand) side of the body. Its counterpart on the non-racquet-hand side, the Eastern backhand, will be discussed later.

Eastern Forehand Grip

The easiest way to assume an **Eastern forehand grip** is simply to hold the racquet on edge so it is perpendicular to the floor and then "shake hands" with the handle (see Photo 3.1). In the shaking-hands position, the first finger and thumb of the racquet hand should form a "V" along the top of the handle, the point of the "V" lying on the midline of the handle's surface (see Photo 3.2). The fingers are spread in a "trigger" position to allow for better wrist snap (see Photo 3.3A and B).

Another way to assume this position is to hold the racquet in the non-racquet hand so the racquet again is on edge. Place your racquet hand with fingers spread on the strings of the racquet so the palm is flat against the racquet face (see Photo 3.4). Slide your racquet hand down the racquet until the end of the handle meets the end of your palm, and wrap your fingers around the handle. Again check to see if the "V" formed by your first finger and thumb is pointed properly along the top bevel (surface) of the handle.

Be careful not to grip the racquet so the handle lies perpendicular to your fingers in a "fist" grip, or the wrist snap will be lost (see Photo 3.5). If you turn the racquet over so your palm is pointed toward the ceiling of the court and open your hand, a racquet in the correct position should

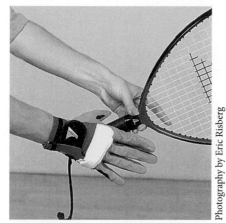

Photography by Eric Risberg

PHOTO 3.1   Shaking Hands with the Racquet.

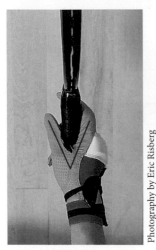

PHOTO 3.2 Eastern Forehand Grip.

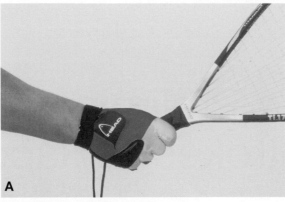

A

Back of Hand

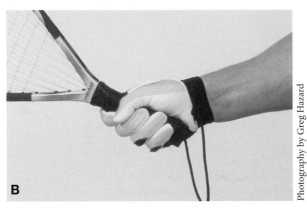

B

Palm of hand

PHOTO 3.3 Trigger Grip.

lie diagonally across the palm (see Photo 3.6). The handle should cover the first knuckle of the first finger and the bottom left side of the palm. The combination of shaking hands, "V" position, and "trigger" finger serve as reminders of an Eastern forehand grip (see Photo 3.7).

Eastern Backhand Grip

If you use the Eastern forehand grip for your forehand shots, you must change your grip to hit backhand shots (shots to the non-racquet-hand side). This is because of the way the arm moves about the elbow. Construction of the elbow joint causes the forearm to move only up and down (flex and extend) when the arm is held straight at your side.

When hitting a backhand shot, the racquet arm is pulled across the body and then extended. If the racquet is held with the forehand grip, the racquet head will be turned up when the ball is hit. Thus, shots that should be hit straight into the front wall will be "popped," or hit up toward the ceiling.

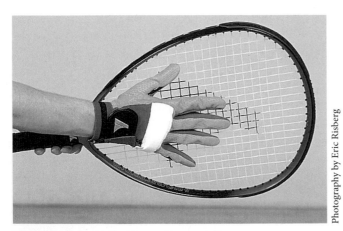

PHOTO 3.4 Palm Flat on Racquet Face.

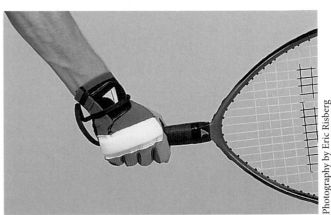

PHOTO 3.5 Improper Grip on Racquet, Fingers Perpendicular to Handle.

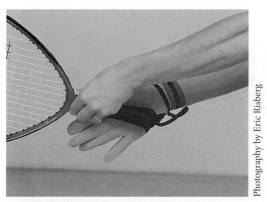

PHOTO 3.6   Handle of Racquet Lying Diagonally Across Palm of Hand.

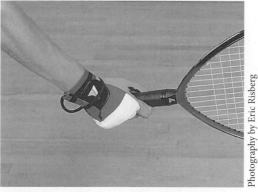

PHOTO 3.7   Assuming the Eastern Forehand Grip.

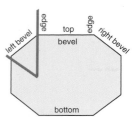

FIGURE 3.1
Racquet Position for Eastern Backhand Grip.

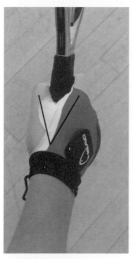

PHOTO 3.8A
Initiation of Change to Eastern Backhand Grip.

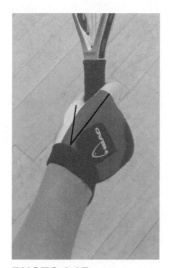

PHOTO 3.8B   The Change to the Eastern Backhand grip, and "V."

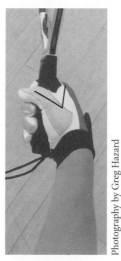

PHOTO 3.8C
Alternative Rotation of Wrist to Hit a Backhand Shot.

To hit a level backhand shot, you must change your grip from the Eastern forehand to the **Eastern backhand grip**. To find this position on your racquet, assume the forehand grip just discussed and hold the racquet on edge. With your non-racquet hand, turn the top of the racquet toward the fingers of your gripping hand so the forefinger–thumb "V" falls on the top left bevel of the racquet (see Figure 3.1). This grip rotates the head of the racquet downward to compensate for the elbow's inability to rotate and allows you to hit a level ball (see Photos 3.8A and 3.8B).

The problem with changing from the forehand grip to the backhand grip is that it takes *time*. Thus, you will have to recognize immediately when you should hit a backhand shot, to give you as much time as possible to make the switch.

A similar situation occurs after taking the backhand shot. The grip must be changed back to the forehand placement. Unfortunately, many players have difficulty changing grips and hitting the ball too! But a player must do something to change the angle of the racquet head.

One alternative solution is to simply rotate the wrist toward the floor when hitting a backhand shot. This turns the racquet head downward and allows a flat shot to be hit (see Photo 3.8C). Returning to the Eastern forehand grip takes only a twist of the wrist. The major problem with this method is that it is so easy that new players often *forget* to do it!

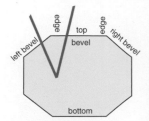

FIGURE 3.2
Continental Grip, and
"V."

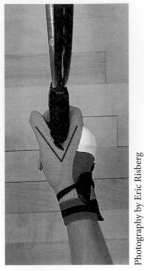

PHOTO 3.9
Continental Grip,
and "V."

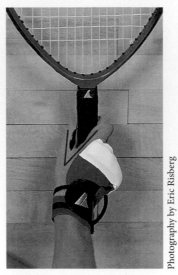

PHOTO 3.10   Western
Grip, Front View.

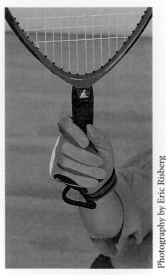

PHOTO 3.11   Western
Grip, Back View.

Either way of changing the racquet position for a backhand shot can be effective as long as you use it consistently. Choose one method and practice it all the time.

Continental Grip

A second alternative to changing grips is to avoid using the Eastern forehand and backhand grips completely. Instead, use the **Continental grip**. In the Continental grip, the racquet is held in a position midway between the Eastern forehand and backhand. To assume this grip, the racquet must be rotated clockwise one-eighth of a turn from the Eastern forehand grip. Now the "V" will point to the top left edge of the handle (see Figure 3.2). Thus, with the Continental grip, little or no adjustment must be made for either a forehand or a backhand shot, although the wrist may be slightly rotated clockwise to adjust the face of the racquet during a backhand shot to hit a level ball (see Photo 3.9).

Western Grip

The third grip, called the **Western grip** or "frying pan" grip (see Photos 3.10 and 3.11), is similar to the grip you use on a frying pan handle when you lift the pan off a stove or pick up your racquet off the floor. Some players prefer this grip for overhead forehand shots, but it is not necessary to change to this grip at all if you are not hitting an overhead shot. The Western grip never should be used to hit a forehand or a backhand shot.

After hitting a few balls, recheck your grip to make sure the racquet has not twisted in your hand. Some players even mark the "V" placement of the thumb and forefinger with tape on the racquet's top bevel. This helps to guide the correct hand positioning.

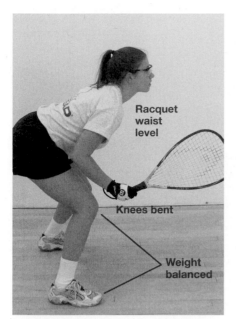

PHOTO 3.12A   Set Position, Side View.

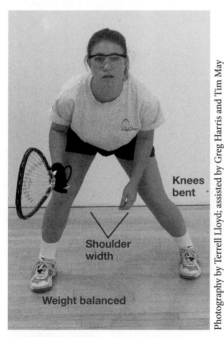

PHOTO 3.12B   Set Position, Front View.

Photography by Terrell Lloyd; assisted by Greg Harris and Tim May

POINTS *to* REMEMBER

Note the position of the "V" on the racquet handle, and make sure it matches your hand placement.

Keep your fingers spread out in a pistol or trigger-finger grip. Don't keep a fist grip on the handle.

Change to a backhand grip or compensate for the elbow's movement by rotating the wrist to hit a ball on the non-racquet side. After taking the shot, change back to a forehand grip.

Use a Western grip, if desired, to hit overhead shots.

All balls can be hit with the Continental grip.

Set, Pivot, and Stroke

The Set

The **set** or "ready" position prepares you to hit the ball. Begin each stroke at the set position and return to it following each hit. The set position allows you to move quickly to hit a ball with either your forehand or your backhand.

To get in the set position, stand with your feet shoulder-width apart, toes pointing forward, and weight equally balanced on the balls of the feet. Hold the racquet in front of you at waist level, and use a forehand grip. Your non-racquet hand should be free to provide ease of movement. The knees should be slightly bent and pointed forward. Shoulders, head, and neck are relaxed, with your eyes free to follow the movement of the ball (see Photos 3.12A and 3.12B). Breathing must be deep and regular.

POINTS *to* REMEMBER

Face the front wall with toes pointed forward.

Balance the weight equally on the balls of the feet, placed shoulder-width apart.

Hold the racquet with a forehand grip in front of you at waist level.

Bend knees and relax head, shoulders, and neck—and the body is ready to spring into action.

The Pivot

As soon as you have decided if the ball is to be hit with a forehand or a backhand stroke, you must **pivot**, or turn your body to prepare for the hit. The sooner the decision can be made, the better prepared you will be to hit the ball. So decide *quickly*. The importance of the pivot is that it turns the hips sideways to the front wall. This allows the player to step into the ball and add his or her body weight into the power of the stroke (see Photos 3.13 and 3.14).

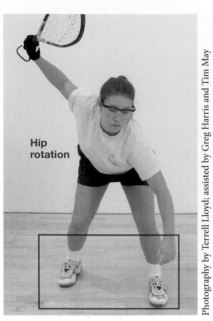

Photography by Terrell Lloyd; assisted by Greg Harris and Tim May

Hip rotation

PHOTO 3.13   Pivot Position for Forehand Stroke.

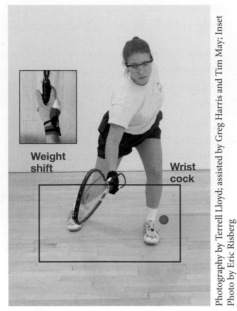

Photography by Terrell Lloyd; assisted by Greg Harris and Tim May; Inset Photo by Eric Risberg

Weight shift

Wrist cock

PHOTO 3.14   Shifting Weight into Ball from Pivot Position for Forehand Stroke.

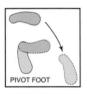

FIGURE 3.3 Forward Pivot for Forehand Stroke.

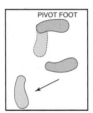

PIVOT FOOT

FIGURE 3.4 Backstep Pivot for Forehand Stroke.

A baseball batter takes the same position. Except to bunt, the batter stands sideways to the pitcher and steps into the pitch by shifting his or her weight forward. Thus, the ball can be hit with more force. Similarly, the pivot in racquetball positions you to step into the ball, shift your weight, and increase the power of your stroke. This is especially important for players who have weaker arms and wrists.

The pivot may be done by moving either forward or back. In either case, you must shift your weight to one foot to turn and face a side wall. Your free foot will be pulled either forward or behind you to complete the pivot. Your body should finish the pivot with your hips facing a side wall.

Whether you step forward or backward when you pivot depends on where the ball rebounds and whether you have to move up or back to reach it (see Figures 3.3 and 3.4). Further adjustments in body position can be made by "cross-stepping" or sliding forward or backward. During any pivot motion, your eyes must not lose contact with the ball and your face should be directed toward the ball.

POINTS *to* REMEMBER

Decide quickly where the ball is to be hit, and pivot to that side immediately.

After the pivot, be sure your body faces a side wall.

Move either forward or backward to the ball by cross-stepping or sliding up or back.

Keep your eyes and face directed at the ball.

Forehand Stroke

The only challenge remaining is to hit the ball! **Forehand** strokes will be discussed first, followed by information on backhand strokes. The forehand stroke itself begins as the racquet is carried from the set stance through the change in position that results from the pivot.

Backswing

As the body is turned to the side wall, so is the racquet. But the racquet continues to be pulled

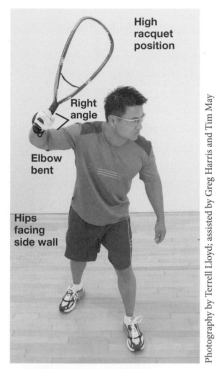

Photography by Terrell Lloyd; assisted by Greg Harris and Tim May

PHOTO 3.15   Completed Backswing with Racquet in Line Between Back Wall and Body.

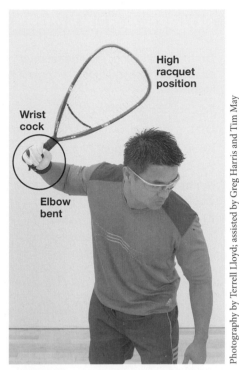

Photography by Terrell Lloyd; assisted by Greg Harris and Tim May

PHOTO 3.16   Wrist Cock on Backswing.

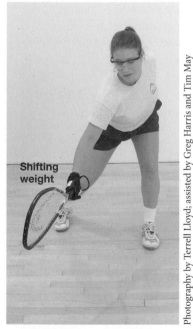

Photography by Terrell Lloyd; assisted by Greg Harris and Tim May

PHOTO 3.17   Weight Shifted Forward to Contact Ball.

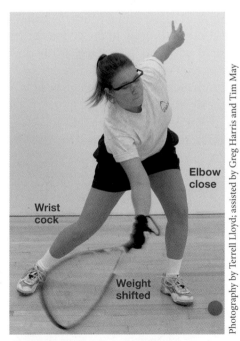

Photography by Terrell Lloyd; assisted by Greg Harris and Tim May

PHOTO 3.18   Forward Swing Maintaining Wrist Cock for Forehand Stroke.

back, so with the elbow bent, the racquet is in a line between your body and the back wall and held high above the head (see Photo 3.15). This is called the **backswing**. In this position the racquet is held almost at a right angle to the forearm, which serves to cock the wrist (see Photo 3.16).

Wrist Cock

The **wrist cock** is a crucial part of your stroke. The uncocking, or snapping, of the wrist and racquet at the ball is what generates the speed and power of the stroke, similarly to throwing a baseball or skipping a rock. Without cocking the wrist there would be no way of hitting the ball with explosive force (see Photo 3.16). To be most effective, the wrist must snap or uncock at the time the ball is contacted.

Forward Swing

As you prepare to swing the racquet forward, you first must shift your weight forward (see Photo 3.17). This is done by stepping into the path of the ball with the foot closest to the front wall. During the swing the elbow must remain close to the side of the body. This position enables the ball to be contacted below waist level and prevents "over-the-shoulder" shots.

The racquet hand should lead the racquet through the swing. This position helps to maintain a cocked wrist during the swing (see Photo 3.18). The elbow should remain bent until the ball is contacted.

At that point, the elbow is extended, the arm is straightened, and the racquet head is snapped forward to meet the ball. Once the arm is extended, the racquet should be at the same level off the floor as your hand, with the head perpendicular to the floor, or "on edge."

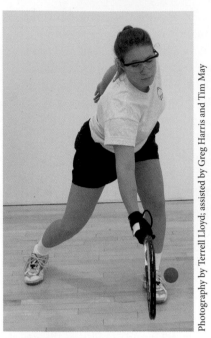

PHOTO 3.19   Contact Point for Forehand Stroke.

Photography by Terrell Lloyd; assisted by Greg Harris and Tim May

---

POINTS *to* REMEMBER

On the backswing, pull the racquet back with the elbow bent to a point directly behind you in line with your body and the back wall, racquet held high.

To cock the wrist, hold the racquet almost at a right angle to the forearm.

On the forward swing, shift the weight to your forward foot.

Keep the elbow bent on the forward swing; hold the upper arm close to the body.

Maintain wrist cock through the swing, with the racquet head trailing the wrist and elbow through the swing.

At the point of contact, extend the arm, keep the racquet head perpendicular to the floor at the same level as the hand, and snap the racquet head forward to meet the ball.

Contact

Contact with the ball should be made opposite your forward foot as your weight shifts forward. At the point of impact, snap the wrist. In most cases, contact with the ball should be as close to the floor as possible, with your arm extended. To do this, you must bend your knees to drop your waist and racquet close to the floor.

You should not drop the racquet below the level of the hand to hit a low ball, nor should you bend from your waist. Your whole body must lower to ensure that the racquet head remains on edge and moves parallel to the ground (see Photo 3.19).

The ball can be contacted at one of three points during its flight (with reference to Figure 3.5): (1) as it rebounds off the front wall, dropping below your waist toward the floor; (2) after the ball rebounds off the floor and bounces toward your racquet; and (3) after the ball reaches the height of

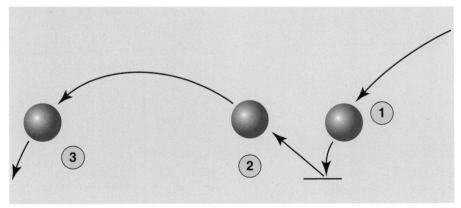

FIGURE 3.5   Points of Contact for a Rebounding Ball.

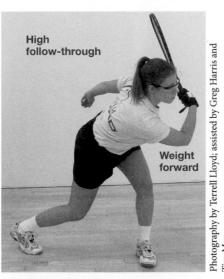

High follow-through

Weight forward

Photography by Terrell Lloyd; assisted by Greg Harris and Tim May

PHOTO 3.20   Follow-through of Forehand Stroke.

its bounce and is falling back to the floor and below your waist.

For experienced players, hitting the ball as it rebounds off the floor (point 2) maintains a fast tempo in the game. Beginning players, however, should wait for the ball to reach the height of its bounce and begin to fall back to the floor for the second time (point 3) before hitting the ball.

> ### POINTS *to* REMEMBER
>
> **Shift** your weight onto your forward foot during the forward swing.
>
> **Hit** the ball opposite your forward foot.
>
> **At** the point of impact, snap the wrist and extend the arm.
>
> **If** possible, contact the ball low to the ground by bending your knees and lowering your body to the ball.

Follow-through

A mistake that many beginners make is failing to complete the stroke, or to follow through, after the hit is made. Consequently, these players punch at the ball with a shortened stroke and lose the force of their hit. The follow-through made after contact with the ball allows for completing the stroke and hitting the ball with all the force of your swing. It also allows you to recover from the stroke quickly and adjust your stance back to the set position to await your next hit.

In general, a racquetball stroke should end with the racquet swung past the midline of the body and finishing high off the non-racquet side. The follow-through should rotate the shoulders and hips so they again are facing the front wall, with the front foot acting as a pivot.

At the end of the stroke, your weight should be concentrated on your forward foot, but balanced so you do not fall down.

During this follow-through, the body should be kept low to the ground (see Photo 3.20). Standing up too quickly will cause the ball to be carried upward with your movement and make it difficult for you to hit low balls. The forehand stroke should follow smoothly in sequential order (see Photo 3.21A–E).

> ### POINTS *to* REMEMBER
>
> **Finish** the stroke with the racquet swung past the midline of the body.
>
> **Stay** low, but allow high racquet follow-through.
>
> **After** the ball has been contacted, allow the body to rotate toward the front wall back to the set position following the direction of the arm swing.
>
> **Don't** stand up until the follow-through is complete.

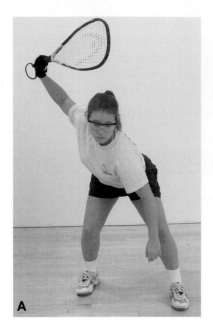

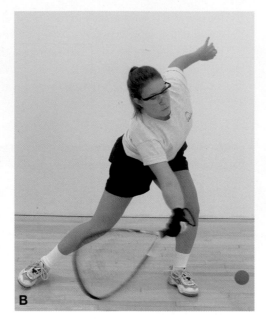

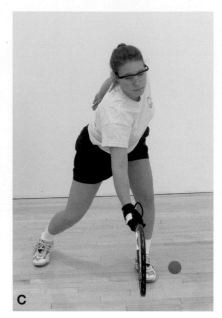

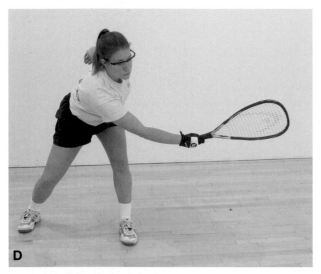

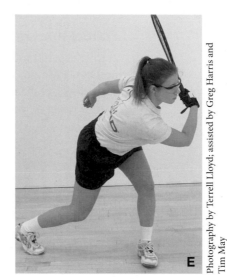

PHOTO 3.21
Forehand Drive
Sequence.

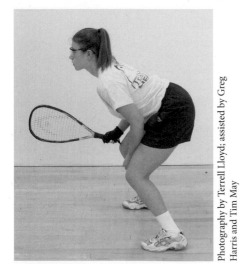

PHOTO 3.22   Set Position, Facing Front Wall.

Backhand Stroke

To hit a **backhand** stroke, use either a backhand grip on the racquet or turn the racquet facedown by rotating the wrist forward. The backhand stroke begins like the forehand stroke from the set position (see Photo 3.22). The pivot, however, results in the player facing the opposite side wall. Again, the pivot can be made by stepping either forward or backward, depending on the position of the ball. After pivoting, the hips should be parallel to the side wall.

Backswing

The backhand stroke is begun by pulling the racquet across the body with the backswing. At the end of the backswing, the racquet is held in line between your shoulder and the back wall with the elbow bent. In this position, the upper body must rotate more than in the forehand stroke for the racquet to be positioned behind the shoulder. When rotated correctly, the chin should almost rest on the shoulder of the racquet arm (see Photo 3.23).

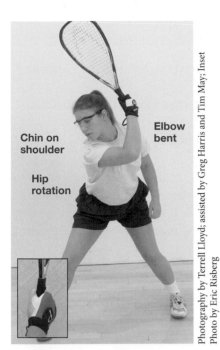

PHOTO 3.23 Backswing Position for Rotation: Chin on Shoulder, Elbow Bent.

Chin on shoulder

Elbow bent

Hip rotation

Photography by Terrell Lloyd; assisted by Greg Harris and Tim May; Inset Photo by Eric Risberg

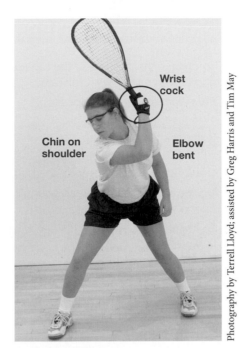

PHOTO 3.24 Wrist Cock for Backhand Stroke.

Wrist cock

Chin on shoulder

Elbow bent

Photography by Terrell Lloyd; assisted by Greg Harris and Tim May

Wrist Cock

The racquet must be held with the wrist cocked, as in the forehand stroke. In the cocked position, the racquet is almost at a 90-degree angle to the forearm (see Photo 3.24).

Forward Swing

As the forward swing is begun, the player's weight is shifted to the front foot. During the forward swing the racquet head should trail the elbow and the hand to maintain the cocked position (see Photos 3.25A and B). The bent elbow should be held close to the body and used as an axis to pivot the racquet around. A common error by a beginning player is to pull the elbow (the "wing") out in front of the body toward the front wall (see Photo 3.26). When this happens, the racquet head is pulled across the body rather than swung directly at the ball, power is lost, and the ball is rebounded to the side of the court.

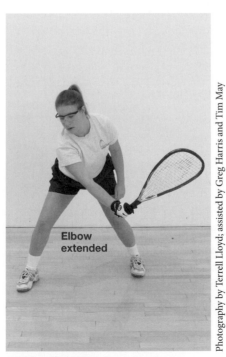

PHOTO 3.25A Cocked Position.

Racquet head trailing elbow

Elbow close to body

PHOTO 3.25B Forward Swing with Racquet Trailing Hand for Backhand Stroke.

Elbow extended

Photography by Terrell Lloyd; assisted by Greg Harris and Tim May

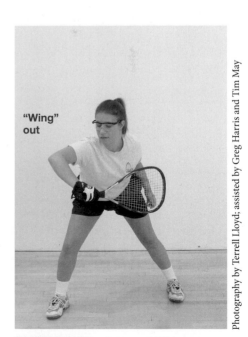

PHOTO 3.26 Incorrect Elbow Position.

"Wing" out

Photography by Terrell Lloyd; assisted by Greg Harris and Tim May

To change the position of the racquet head to hit the ball, use a backhand grip or rotate your wrist forward.

Pivot to the side wall opposite from the wall turned to with the forehand stroke.

Pull back the racquet to a position between the shoulder and the back wall with the elbow bent, racquet held high.

Cock the wrist at the end of the backswing.

On the forward swing, keep your elbow close to the body and pivot the racquet head around it.

To maintain the wrist cock, keep the racquet head behind the hand on the forward swing.

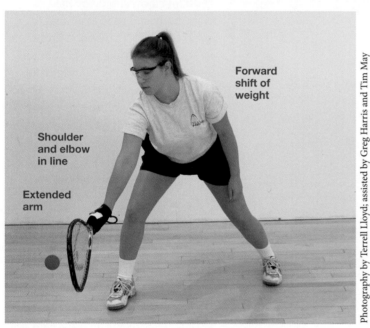

Forward shift of weight

Shoulder and elbow in line

Extended arm

Photography by Terrell Lloyd; assisted by Greg Harris and Tim May

PHOTO 3.27   Contacting the Ball for Backhand Stroke.

Contact

To contact the ball, your weight should be forward on the front foot.

Extend the elbow at the point of contact so the racquet head is now in line with the wrist, elbow, and shoulder. The racquet should contact the ball just opposite the forward foot as low to the ground as possible (see Photo 3.27). When the ball is contacted, the wrist is snapped sharply, similar to throwing a Frisbee, to bring the racquet in line with the hand and thereby increase the impact on the ball.

Shift your weight forward at contact with the ball.

Hit the ball when it is opposite your forward foot and close to the floor.

At the point of contact, extend the arm, keeping the elbow close to the body.

As the racquet hits the ball, snap the wrist to increase the power in your stroke.

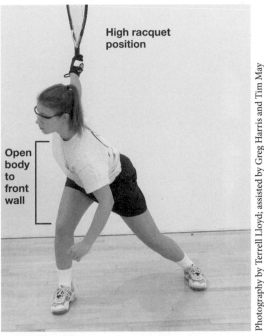

High racquet position

Open body to front wall

Photography by Terrell Lloyd; assisted by Greg Harris and Tim May

PHOTO 3.28   Follow-through on Backhand Stroke.

Follow-through

As with the forehand, the backhand stroke is finished with a **follow-through**.

With the follow-through, the chest and hips end up facing the front wall, and the racquet is swung to a point opposite the shoulder of the racquet arm. Without a follow-through, the strength of the swing is lost.

Until the stroke is complete, keep your head down to prevent yourself from standing up before the ball leaves the racquet (see Photo 3.28). Otherwise the ball will be lifted up with your movement. Similar to the forehand stroke, the backhand stroke should be executed in one smooth motion (see Photos 3.29A–E).

The success of either a forehand or a backhand stroke will depend upon your ability to hit the ball consistently with the same stroking motion. This means that the point of contact with the ball in relation to your body must not vary. The only way to assure this is to *move* on the court so the ball is aligned properly with your stroke.

Too many beginning players (and some better ones, too!) are content to hit the ball regardless of where it is, if it is within their reach. This tactic results in many unorthodox strokes used to hit the ball. Most of these shots have never been practiced, so the strokes are merely rebounding the ball back to the front wall rather than being accurately placed. The player who is consistently positioned to hit a practiced shot can make conscious changes in the racquet head angle or force of impact to *direct* the ball away from the opponent's reach. Now *that* is racquetball!

POINTS *to* REMEMBER

Finish the stroke with a follow-through so the racquet stops at a point opposite the forward shoulder.

Stay low after hitting the ball.

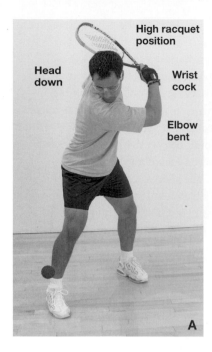

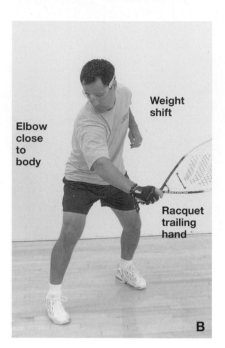

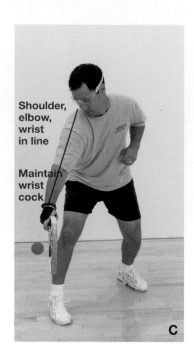

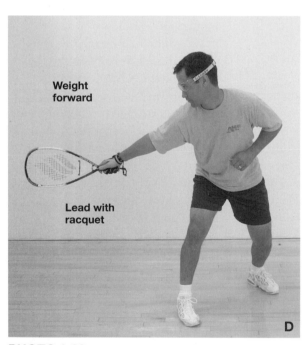

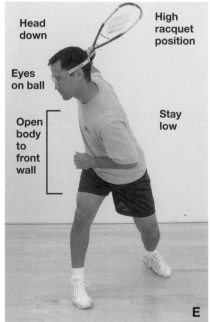

PHOTO 3.29   Backhand Drive Sequence.

Photography by Terrell Lloyd; assisted by Greg Harris and Tim May

COMMON ERRORS **HOW TO CORRECT THEM**

1. I never know where the ball is going.

You fail to position yourself so the ball is contacted at the same place in relation to your body at all times. Move in the court, and go to where the ball will be. Set yourself up, and hit the ball as you have practiced.

2. I can't hit the ball hard.

Check to see if you are following through rather than just punching at the ball and stopping your arm motion.

Make sure your wrist is cocked and you are snapping your wrist at the moment of contact with the ball to increase the impact.

Make sure you are hitting the ball when you shift your weight forward.

3. The ball always goes up. I can't seem to hit a low ball.

Check your grip to see if the racquet head is pointed up at contact.

Watch your body position to see if you are standing up before the ball leaves the racquet head. You may be carrying the ball up with you.

Emphasize a low follow-through rather than just punching at the ball.

Let the ball drop lower before you hit it, and keep the racquet perpendicular to the floor.

4. I miss the ball completely, or the ball always hits a side wall first.

You probably are hitting the ball off your back foot. This area is not in your field of vision, and you lose track of the ball. Hitting the ball from this position also means that your arm has not swung the racquet far enough so the racquet head is parallel to the front wall at contact. Instead, the racquet head is still angled toward a side wall, causing the ball to rebound in that direction.

5. I hit the ball into the side wall.

Usually this means you have not changed from the set position to the pivot. Your hips therefore are facing the front wall rather than the side wall. As a result, your stroke comes across the body and directs the ball into the side wall.

If it is a backhand shot, you also may be pulling your elbow in front of your body rather than pivoting around it during the swing.

You could be hitting off your back foot. See answer 4.

6. I can't hit my backhand with strength and power.

You are positioning yourself too close to the ball on your backhand side. As a result, you cannot extend your arm and utilize the wrist snap at the point of contact to maximize your power.

CHECKPOINTS

Answers are located on page 141.

1. The Eastern forehand grip is characterized by:
   a. a shake-hands position on the grip with a V formed by the index finger and thumb on top of the grip, and a trigger-finger position on the grip.
   b. a shake-hands position on the top of the grip with a V formed by the finger and thumb on top of the grip, and a grip with the fingers perpendicular to the handle.
   c. a shake-hands position on the grip with a V formed by the index finger and thumb pointed to the racquet-side shoulder, and a trigger-finger position on the grip.
   d. a fist grip with fingers perpendicular to the handle.

2. The position of the V formed by the index finger and thumb when using a Continental grip is positioned:
   a. with the V pointed toward the bottom left edge of the handle.
   b. with the V pointed toward the top left edge of the handle.
   c. with the V pointed toward the bottom center of the handle.

   d. with the V pointed toward the top right edge of the handle.

3. The Western grip is used to hit:
   a. forehand shots.
   b. backhand shots.
   c. both types of shots.
   d. neither type of shot.

4. The set position requires:
   a. a racquet position at waist level and knees bent with weight forward.
   b. a racquet position at waist level and knees bent with weight balanced.
   c. a racquet position at waist level and knees extended with weight balanced.
   d. a racquet position at waist level and knees extended with weight forward.

5. The critical part of a racquetball stroke is:
   a. a wrist cock followed by a snap of the wrist at contact.
   b. a firm wrist followed by a sweeping motion at contact.
   c. a firm wrist followed by a snap of the wrist at contact.
   d. a wrist cock followed by a sweeping motion at contact.

6. The follow-through when executing a racquetball basic stroke is characterized by:
   a. the racquet and body finishing high with balance on the lead foot.
   b. the racquet finishing high with the body staying low and balance on the lead foot.
   c. the racquet finishing high with the body staying low and balance on the back foot.
   d. the racquet and body finishing high and balance on the back foot.

7. The correction required to eliminate hitting a basic stroke into the side wall first before hitting the front wall is to:
   a. pivot from the set position so your hips are facing the side wall.
   b. make contact with the ball off your lead foot.
   c. neither a nor b.
   d. both a and b.

8. When making contact with the ball, the body position should include:
   a. stepping away from the ball.
   b. stepping into the ball.
   c. neither a nor b.
   d. both a and b, in sequence.

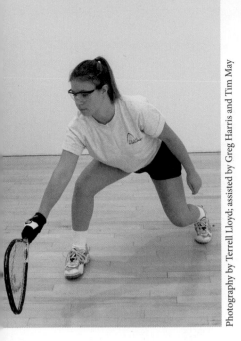

Photography by Terrell Lloyd; assisted by Greg Harris and Tim May

Offensive Strokes

An **offensive shot** is designed to win a point outright by virtue of the skill with which it is hit. Regardless of where your opponent is playing, the well-executed offensive shot should always be a winner. There are several basic offensive shots. Any offensive shot may be hit with either a forehand or a backhand stroke, and the skilled player can use either stroke with equal effectiveness.

The beginning player usually will choose to hit an offensive shot from the forehand side. This gives credence to the observation of a player having a "weak" side (one from which an offensive shot is usually not hit—in most cases—the backhand). Therefore, a good strategy to follow when playing a *weak-sided* opponent is to hit your offensive shots so they must be returned with a "weak" side shot (backhand). With this strategy, if your offensive shot is not perfect, you are usually not setting up an offensive return.

The type of offensive shot you hit depends upon your skill with each shot, your position on the court, and, in a few instances, your opponent's court position. To hit accurate offensive shots requires hours of practice on the court. Therefore, you should not rely on offensive shots in a game situation until you can hit them consistently in practice.

Kill Shots

A **kill shot** is the ultimate offensive weapon of a racquetball player. By definition, a kill shot is a ball that hits the front wall so low and hard that the rebound to the floor occurs almost simultaneously with the front-wall hit (see Figure 4.1). This rebound makes it virtually impossible for your opponent to return the ball even if he or she is standing in the ball's path.

All kill shots except the overhead kill should be hit when the ball is close to the floor. Contact with the ball must be made by bending your knees to drop your waist and racquet arm close to the floor. Ideally, the ball should be struck when it is positioned between your bent knee and the top of your foot (see Photos 4.1 and 4.2). The shot then is made with a normal forehand or backhand motion, with emphasis on generating power in the hit by stepping into the ball and using a good wrist snap (see Photos 4.3A–E and 4.4A–E).

The harder the ball is hit, the farther away from the front wall a kill shot can be successfully made. Most

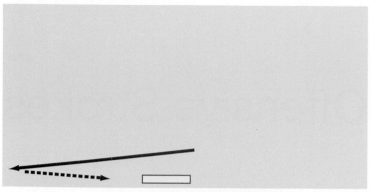

FIGURE 4.1 Rebound of a Kill shot off Front Wall.

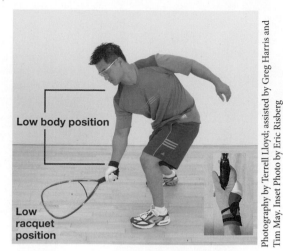

Photography by Terrell Lloyd; assisted by Greg Harris and Tim May. Inset Photo by Eric Risberg

PHOTO 4.1 Forehand Racquet Position to Hit Kill Shot.

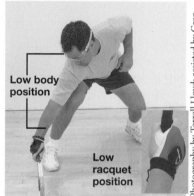

PHOTO 4.2 Backhand Racquet Position to Hit Kill Shot.

Photography by Terrell Lloyd; assisted by Greg Harris and Tim May. Inset Photo by Greg Hazard

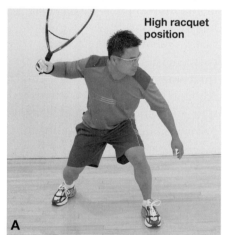

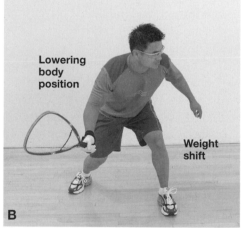

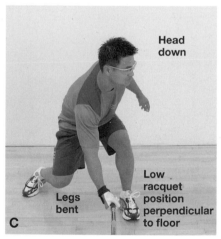

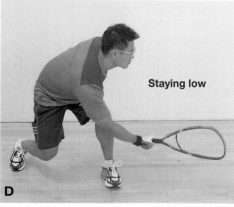

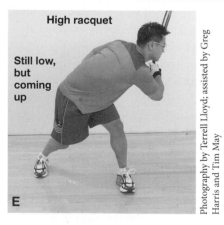

Photography by Terrell Lloyd; assisted by Greg Harris and Tim May

PHOTO 4.3 Forehand Kill Shot Sequence.

beginners, however, because of their weaker stroke, should concentrate on hitting kill shots from a midcourt position or just behind the short line.

The critical factor in hitting a good kill shot is keeping the racquet perpendicular to the floor and the swing parallel to the floor to ensure hitting a flat or level ball. A level hit will rebound off the front wall at or below the height that it hits into the wall. Thus, a low, level ball hit to the

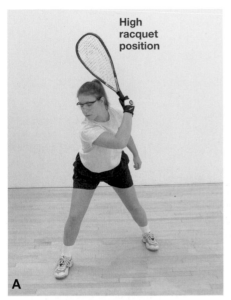

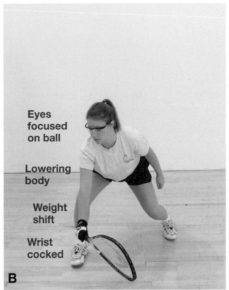

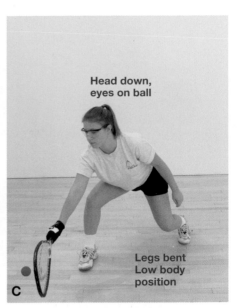

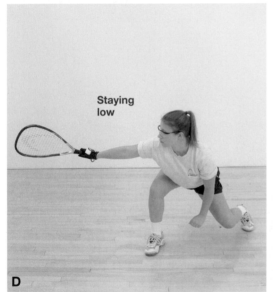

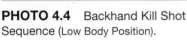

PHOTO 4.4 Backhand Kill Shot Sequence (Low Body Position).

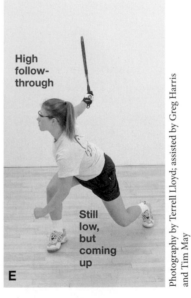

Photography by Terrell Lloyd; assisted by Greg Harris and Tim May

front wall has the greatest potential for achieving the desired kill shot effect (see Photo 4.5A–C).

Front Wall–Straight-In Kill Shot

A **front wall–straight-in kill shot** hits the front wall first and rebounds toward the back wall without touching a side wall. This shot can be hit from anyplace in the court and at any time during play, but it is most effective if your opponent is (A) next to or (B) behind you in the court (see Figure 4.2).

Ideally, this kill shot should be directed toward the half of the front wall farthest from the opposing player. Because the ball follows a straight path to the front wall, the racquet face must be parallel to this surface when it strikes the ball. In addition, keeping the swing level to the floor will ensure that the ball is hit low to the front wall.

Front Wall–Side Wall Kill Shot to the Corner

As shown in Figure 4.3, if the opponent is (A) close to a side wall or (B) in the back court, a corner kill shot may be used. In this shot, the racquet is held so that at the point of contact, the ball is aimed at a corner of the front wall (see Photo 4.6). As a result, the ball will hit the front wall close to a front wall–side wall corner and quickly rebound to the nearest side wall.

Depending upon the angle at which the ball is hit, the ball may bounce toward a front- or a midcourt position. The success of this shot depends on your opponent's court position and how accurately you can

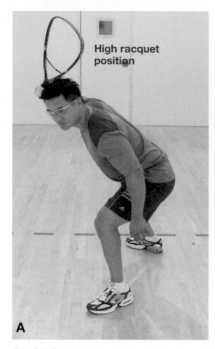

High racquet position

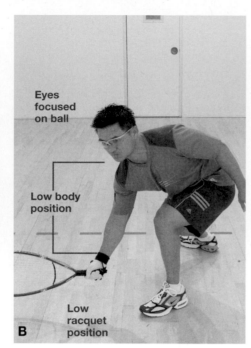

Eyes focused on ball

Low body position

Low racquet position

A   **B**

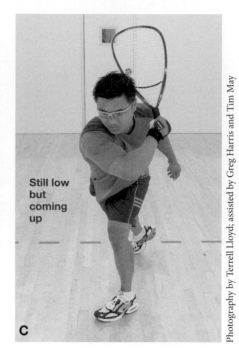

Still low but coming up

C

Photography by Terrell Lloyd; assisted by Greg Harris and Tim May

PHOTO 4.5   Form for a Forehand Kill Shot.

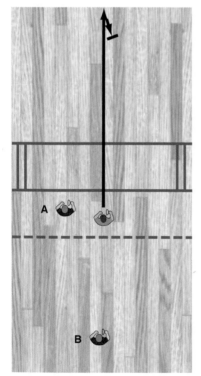

A

B

FIGURE 4.2   Front Wall–Straight-in Kill Shot.

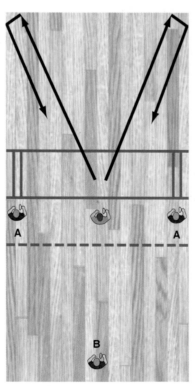

A   A

B

FIGURE 4.3   Front Wall–Side Wall Kill to Corner.

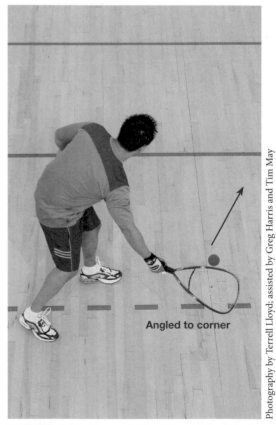

Angled to corner

Photography by Terrell Lloyd; assisted by Greg Harris and Tim May

PHOTO 4.6   Racquet Head Angled to Front Corner for Kill Shot.

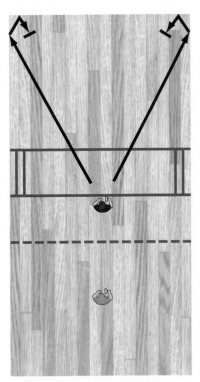

FIGURE 4.4 Side Wall–Front Wall Kill (Pinch).

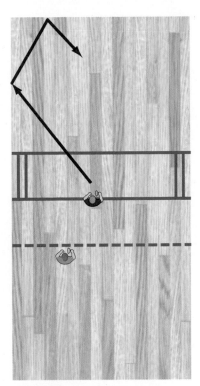

FIGURE 4.5 Pinch Kill Hit Away from Opponent.

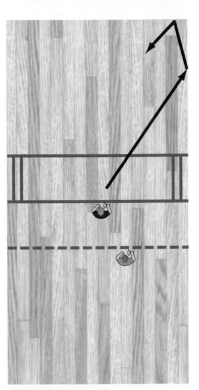

FIGURE 4.6 Pinch Kill Hit to Opponent's Backhand.

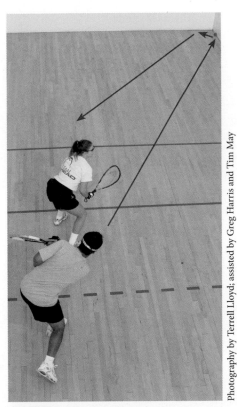

PHOTO 4.7 Pinch Kill Hit to Opponent's Weak Side.

Photography by Terrell Lloyd; assisted by Greg Harris and Tim May

hit the ball. If the ball is not hit low as a kill shot should be, or if the opponent is not far enough in the back court or toward a side wall, the shot will be a set up for an easy return to the front wall. One way to adjust for a quick-reacting opponent who covers the court well is to hit the corner kill at a sharper angle closer to the corner so that the ball rebounds toward the front-court position.

Side Wall–Front Wall Kill Shot (Pinch)

The **pinch kill shot** hits one side wall before rebounding into the front wall. An advantage of hitting the pinch kill rather than the corner kill is simply the placement of the rebounding ball. Where the corner kill is more likely to rebound close to a midcourt position, the pinch kill rebounds tightly into the front court (see Figure 4.4). To be most effective with the pinch kill, the opponent should be next to or behind you in the court.

Whether the shot is directed to the left or to the right front corner depends partly on your position in the court but, more importantly, on your opponent's position. Ideally, you should always hit the ball so that the rebound off the front wall is traveling away from the opponent (see Figure 4.5). If this can't be done, at least hit the ball so that it rebounds toward the opponent's weak side. A shot to the weak side, even if not perfectly hit, should not result in an offensive return (see Figure 4.6 and Photo 4.7).

To hit a pinch kill (as with the corner kill), the racquet face upon contact with the ball must be angled to the side wall rather than held parallel to the front wall. The ball must be contacted close to the ground. To do this, bend your knees, drop your waist, and extend your racquet arm down (see Photo 4.6). In all other

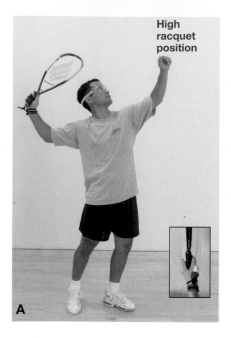

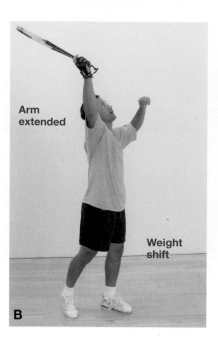

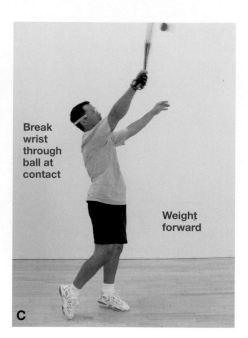

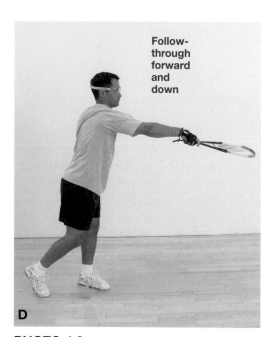

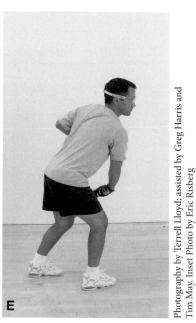

PHOTO 4.8   Forehand overhead kill shot sequence.

Photography by Terrell Lloyd; assisted by Greg Harris and Tim May. Inset Photo by Eric Risberg

respects, the technique for hitting this kill shot is similar to that for a forehand or backhand stroke (see Photos 3.21 and 3.29 in Chapter 3).

The pinch kill is ideal for beginning players because they can make a mistake in hitting this shot and still score a point. Because the rebound is to a front-court position, even a ball hit too high or one that rebounds off the floor may be impossible for your opponent to reach as long as he or she is in the back court.

Overhead Kill

The **overhead kill shot** is popular with beginning players but falls out of favor as the player develops other offensive weapons. The object of the overhead kill is the same as for any kill shot, but the stroking technique is different. This kill shot is hit from a ball that is above shoulder level rather than close to the floor. It is hit from the forehand side with a motion similar to a tennis serve (see Photo 4.8A–E). The stroke is begun by pulling the racquet back as if to hit a forehand stroke. As the forward swing is begun, however, the racquet is lifted in a circular motion as if you were going to throw it to the front wall. The chest and hips are rotated to face the front wall as you step forward to hit the ball. The ball is contacted just in front of the forward foot with an extended arm.

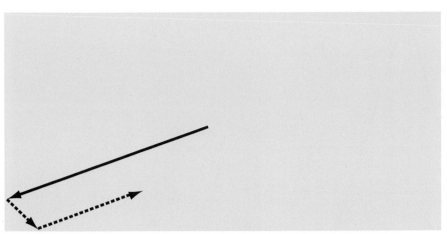

FIGURE 4.7 Rebound of Poorly Hit Overhead Kill Bouncing High Off Floor.

snap. Complete the stroke with a follow-through, bringing the racquet through the ball toward the target.

Ideally, the ball should be directed low into the front corner of the court. To have the best chance of success, the overhead kill should hit a side wall as well as the front wall to deaden the rebound of the ball. Otherwise, if not hit perfectly, the ball will rebound high into the air at the same angle at which it hit the wall (see Figure 4.7). The high bounce gives even slow opponents adequate time to position themselves for the return. Consequently, the overhead kill is considered a "low-percentage" shot because it is hard to score a point off a ball that is not hit perfectly.

Beginning players are advised to be patient and wait for the ball to drop below waist level rather than hit an overhead kill. Then a corner or pinch kill can be hit.

Both of these kill shots are more difficult to return than the overhead kill, even if they are hit incorrectly.

At contact, the face of the racquet should be angled slightly down to the front wall. To assume this position, a Western grip is preferred over any other forehand grip in order to point the face of the racquet to the front wall. To maximize the power of the stroke, the ball should always be hit with the arm in an extended position with a downward wrist

POINTS to REMEMBER

To hit an effective kill shot, wait for the ball to fall low to the floor—at least below your knee.

To reach the ball, pivot, bend your knees, and drop your waist to lower your racquet arm toward the ground.

To hit a straight-in kill shot, keep your racquet face perpendicular to the floor and parallel to the front wall. Swing level with the floor using a good wrist snap.

To direct a kill shot to a front corner, angle your racquet face to the corner that you wish to hit.

Try to angle your kill shot away from your opponent's court position or hit to his or her weak side to ensure a successful shot.

Passing Shots

A **passing shot**, unlike the kill shot, requires no new techniques to master.

Its effectiveness depends only on your opponent's court position and your ability to place the ball.

The passing shot, as its name implies, is a ball that literally goes past the opponent. Therefore, it is most advantageous to hit when the opposing player is in the front-, mid-, or center-court areas. In this way, the ball can go past the opponent and

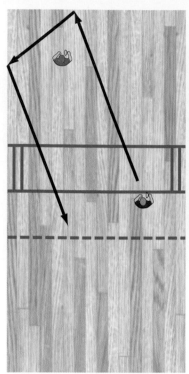

FIGURE 4.8   Passing Shot Hit when Opponent is Caught in Front Court.

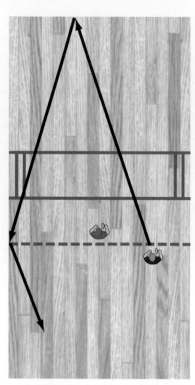

FIGURE 4.9   Passing Shot Hit When Opponent is Positioned in Center Court.

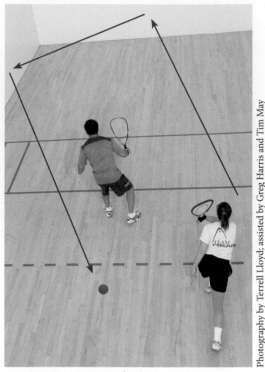

PHOTO 4.9   Passing Shot Hitting Side Wall at Same Distance from Front Wall that Opponent is Standing.

Photography by Terrell Lloyd; assisted by Greg Harris and Tim May

beat him or her into the back court (see Figures 4.8 and 4.9).

If hit low off the front wall, a passing shot will die in the back court and not rebound into a center-court position. Without rebounding hard off the back wall, the ball is, in essence, out-of-play, except to a heroic effort. At the very least, if the ball is returned, it usually will be a desperation shot that you can return for a winner, or it will push your opponent to use up his or her energy reserves.

The most critical error beginning players make when using a passing shot is to hit the ball with too much force. As a result, instead of dying in the back court, the ball rebounds off the back wall into play and negates the advantage the passing shot offers.

The passing shot can be hit with a forehand, a backhand, or an overhead stroke. The ball should be directed to hit the front wall at a point between waist and knee height off the floor.

In all cases, however, the lower the rebound off the front wall, the less is the chance that a return will be made.

The ball can be hit directly to a back corner, or it can be angled to rebound from the front wall to contact a side wall on the way to the back court. If the ball is angled toward a side wall, it should hit at the same distance or farther from the front wall as your opponent is standing (see Photo 4.9). This will help to slow the movement of the ball into the back court and also discourage your opponent from trying to hit the ball as it rebounds off the front wall, because it will be out of reach.

If the ball hits the side wall in front of your opponent's court position, it will pass through the center court and allow your opponent to make a play on the ball.

Two types of passing shots are common: the down-the-line pass and the cross-court pass.

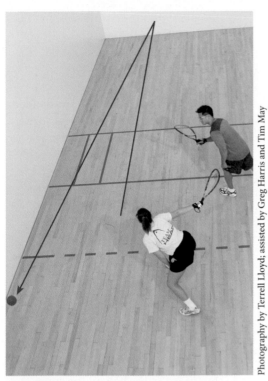

PHOTO 4.10 Down-the-line Pass.

Photography by Terrell Lloyd; assisted by Greg Harris and Tim May

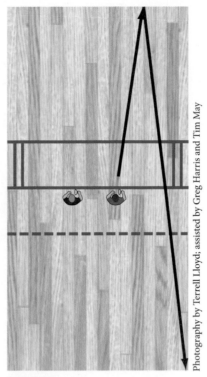

FIGURE 4.10 Down-the-line Pass.

Photography by Terrell Lloyd; assisted by Greg Harris and Tim May

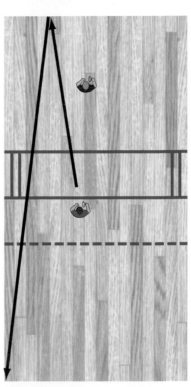

FIGURE 4.11 Passing Shot to Weak Side When Opponent is in Front Court.

Down-the-Line Pass

The **down-the-line** pass could really be called the down-the-wall (wallpaper) pass. This ball is hit so it travels in a line along the side wall, one to three feet from it and below waist level (see Photo 4.10). As stated before, hitting the ball too hard will cause a strong rebound off the back wall and possibly allow a return to be made. This passing shot ideally is hit when you are between your opponent and the side wall down which you are hitting, or when the opposing player is caught off guard in a front-court position (see Figures 4.10 and 4.11).

In either case, hit the ball toward the side wall that is the farthest distance from your opponent. If he or she is playing a center-court position, hit to the backhand side. Use a forehand stroke to hit down-the-line passing shots to the forehand side of the court and a backhand stroke for balls directed to the backhand side.

Cross-Court Pass

The **cross-court pass** moves the ball from one side of the court to the other side in order to pass the opponent. It does this by following the path of a "V" across the court (see Figures 4.12 and 4.13). Depending upon where you are positioned in the court, the ball will rebound off the front wall close to its center.

You must experiment with the exact placement of the ball as you hit from different court positions.

What will always be true is that the ball will rebound from the front wall at an angle equal to the angle of impact. To prevent the opponent from hitting the rebound off the front wall, this angle must be great enough to avoid the opponent's reach.

As with a down-the-line pass, the cross-court shot may be hit with a forehand, a backhand, or an overhead stroke. Ideally, it is used when your opponent is forward on your

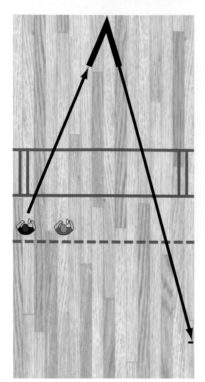

FIGURE 4.12 Cross-court Passing Shot with Opponent Close to Side Wall.

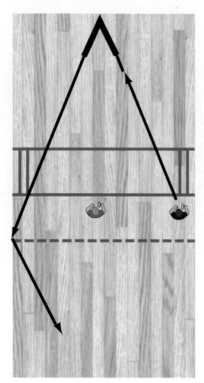

FIGURE 4.13 Cross-court Passing Shot with Opponent in Center Court.

side of the court, is in a center-court position, or is positioned closer to a side wall.

One advantage of the cross-court passing shot is that it can be hit from anyplace on the court, including the back court, as the success of the shot depends on your opponent's court position.

It is an easy shot to learn and win with because most right-handed players can use their stronger forehands to hit cross-court passing shots to their opponents' weaker backhands.

As with a down-the-line pass, a ball that rebounds low into the back court has the greatest chance for success. This ball also may hit a side wall before rebounding into the back-court area (see Figure 4.13). As stated earlier, however, care must be taken to ensure that the ball does not rebound through a center-court position or in front of the opponent. Hitting a side wall also will help to slow the speed of the ball on the court, allowing you to hit the ball with more force and still have a successful passing shot.

Because there is a wide margin of error with how hard and at what angle the ball should be hit, even the beginning player can make successful cross-court passing shots.

POINTS *to* REMEMBER

A passing shot can be hit with any stroke. Its success depends upon your opponent's court position.

A passing shot should not be used when your opponent is in a back-court position.

A passing shot can be hit cross-court or down-the-line from anyplace on the court.

As long as the ball goes into the back court, the lower the passing shot rebounds off the front wall, the greater is its chance of being a winning shot.

The passing shot may hit a side wall after rebounding from the front wall, but it should not be angled to hit in front of the opponent or to go through the center-court area.

Hitting the passing shot too hard will cause the ball to rebound off the back wall into play.

COMMON ERRORS **HOW TO CORRECT THEM**

1. My kill shots always hit the floor before they reach the front wall.

   You probably have angled the racquet face down at the point of impact with the ball, driving the ball into the floor. Concentrate on keeping your racquet face perpendicular to the floor and the stroke parallel to the floor.

2. My kill shots are never low enough to the front wall.

   Be patient and wait for the ball to drop closer to the floor before hitting it. This means that you will have to bend your knees and lower your waist to drop your racquet to the ball. Try to make contact with the ball just off the tops of your shoes. If this does not help, you may be scooping at the ball with the racquet and hitting it on the upswing, which lifts the ball to the front wall higher than you want it to hit. A level swing with the floor will correct this problem.

3. I hit my cross-court shots right back to my opponent because the ball bounces off a side wall into the center court.

   Take some angle off your hit, and aim more for the center of the front wall.

4. My down-the-line passing shot always hits the side wall.

   The racquet head is not parallel to the front wall when you contact the ball, but instead is angled toward the side wall you are hitting. Snap your wrist and swing through the ball.

   Also, check to make sure you are contacting the ball off your forward foot. Contacting the ball off your back foot can cause the ball to rebound into the side wall after hitting the front wall.

5. My overhead kill shot hits (a) the floor first or (b) too high off the front wall.

   When the floor is hit first, the ball is hit either when it is too far in front of you or when your wrist is bent too much, causing the racquet head to be angled to the floor. Check the position of your body relative to the ball when you hit the overhead, and hold the racquet so it appears to be an extension of your arm.

   Hitting the ball too high off the front wall usually results from hitting the ball too far behind your front foot or even over your head, which prevents you from angling the hit downward. Again, check the position of the ball when you make contact, and be sure that the contact point is in front of your forward foot.

6. My passing shots always rebound off the back wall into a center-court position.

   Take some of the force off your stroke, and hit the ball lower off the front wall to ensure a shorter rebound from the back. If this does not help, try to hit a side wall to deaden the ball's movement.

CHECKPOINTS

Answers located on page 141.

1. A kill shot can best be described as the ultimate offensive weapon that strikes the:
   a. front wall low and hard with the rebound of the ball contacting the floor almost at the same time as the front wall.
   b. front wall at knee level or lower and rebounds low off the wall.
   c. front wall low and hard with the ball rebounding deep to the back wall.
   d. front wall at knee level or lower and rebounds to the back wall.

2. The critical factor in hitting a kill shot is to:
   a. keep the racquet perpendicular to the floor and the swing with the racquet face closed.
   b. keep the racquet perpendicular to the floor and the swing parallel to the floor.
   c. keep the racquet at a 45-degree angle to the floor and the swing with racquet face closed.
   d. keep the racquet at a 45-degree angle to the floor and the swing parallel to the floor.

3. The corner kill combination is:
   a. front wall, side wall.
   b. side wall, front wall.
   c. side wall, back wall.
   d. front wall, back wall.

4. The pinch kill combination is:
   a. front wall, side wall.
   b. side wall, front wall.
   c. side wall, back wall.
   d. both a and b.

5. An overhead kill shot is:
   a. contacted from a high racquet position and the ball strikes the front wall low with a high bounce.
   b. contacted with a high racquet position and the ball strikes the front wall low with the ball contacting the front wall and the floor almost at the same time.
   c. contacted from a high racquet position and the ball strikes the side wall and front wall corner.
   d. contacted from a low racquet position and the ball strikes the front wall and side wall corner.

6. A down-the-line passing shot is hit:
   a. down the side wall 1–3 feet from the wall and above waist level.
   b. down the side wall 1–3 feet from the wall and below waist level.
   c. down the side wall, grazing the wall at below waist level.
   d. down the side wall, grazing the wall at above waist level.

7. A cross-court passing shot:
   a. is hit low, striking the front wall and rebounding in the path of a V.
   b. is hit high, striking the front wall and rebounding in the path of a V.
   c. is hit low, striking the front and side walls in the path of a V.
   d. is hit high, striking the front and side walls in the path of a V.

8. Cross-court passing shots that strike the front and side wall, returning to your opponent, can be corrected by:
   a. hitting with more angle.
   b. hitting with less angle.
   c. aiming more to the center of the front wall.
   d. none of the above.

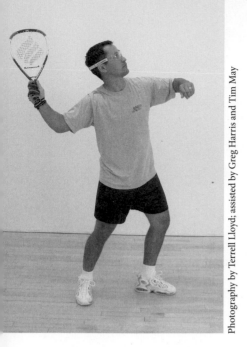

5

Defensive Strokes

Rather than scoring a point, the purpose of a defensive shot is to *prevent* your opponent from hitting a winning shot. This goal can be achieved only if the ball rebounds high off the front wall, preventing a kill-shot return, or rebounds to a court position that does not favor an offensive return. The best defensive shot is hit in such a way as to have the ball rebound from the front wall high into the back court and close to the side wall. Several strokes accomplish this purpose, at least one of which should immediately become part of your repertoire of shots.

Ceiling–Front Wall Shots

A ceiling–front wall shot can be hit with either a forehand or a backhand from any part of the court. A ceiling–front wall shot hits the ceiling before it hits the front wall. Upon contact with the ceiling, the ball rebounds to the front wall close to the ceiling–front wall seam and then is directed downward to bounce on the floor, hitting in front of the service zone before rebounding into the back-court area (see Figure 5.1).

To hit this shot properly, the ball should be directed to hit the ceiling

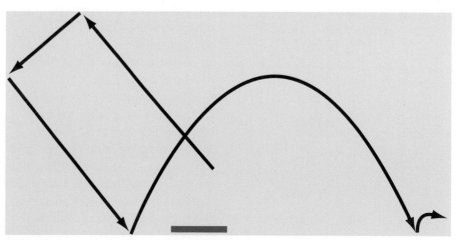

FIGURE 5.1 Ceiling-front wall defensive shot.

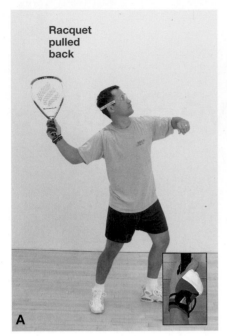

Racquet pulled back

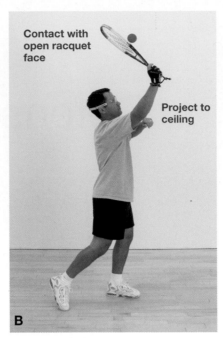

Contact with open racquet face

Project to ceiling

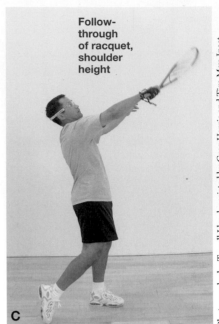

Follow-through of racquet, shoulder height

Photography by Terrell Lloyd; assisted by Greg Harris and Tim May. Inset Photo by Eric Risberg

PHOTO 5.1   Forehand Overhead Ceiling Shot Sequence.

approximately two to three feet from the ceiling–front wall seam. The advantage of a ceiling–front wall shot is that it can be an effective defensive shot even if your opponent is near the center court. This is because the rebound of the ball off the floor will carry it high over the opponent's head and, hopefully, into the back corner.

Because the ball must be returned before striking the floor twice, your opponent must hit the ball from this corner position before the ball touches the floor again. Thus, this court position makes it difficult to hit an offensive shot because of the ball's proximity to the walls.

More importantly, this is an easy shot to learn because the harder you hit the ceiling–front wall shot, the higher the height of the bounce off the floor, and the ball will still land in the back court. Thus, this is not a shot that requires finesse to hit effectively, and it can be used successfully with relatively little practice.

The ceiling–front wall shot is used most typically on a ball that can be hit

with an overhead stroke, either on the forehand (see Photos 5.1A–C) or backhand (see Photos 5.2A–C) side. For this reason, an overhead ceiling–front wall shot is similar in technique to an overhead kill shot (see Chapter 4). Unlike in the kill shot, however, contact with the ball can be made just off the forward foot, with the hips and chest facing the front wall and the arm extended. When hitting a ceiling shot, many players prefer a Western grip, as it opens the face of the racquet to the ceiling.

The difference between the ceiling shot and the offensive kill return is the angle of the racquet face when it contacts the ball. With the ceiling shot, the racquet face must be angled toward the ceiling. To do this, the wrist cannot be snapped from its laid-back position (see Photo 5.3) on the forward swing. This will keep the racquet directed upward. The stroke should finish with a follow-through to ensure hitting the ball with power.

A ceiling–front wall shot also can be hit from a ball that has dropped below waist level. For this shot, the stroke begins like any other forehand

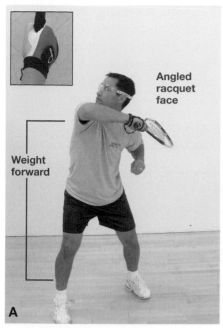

Weight forward

Angled racquet face

A

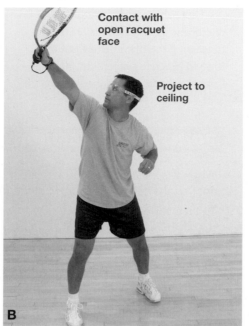

Contact with open racquet face

Project to ceiling

B

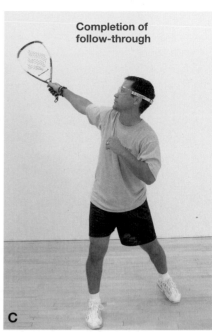

Completion of follow-through

C

Photography by Terrell Lloyd; assisted by Greg Harris and Tim May. Inset Photo by Greg Hazard

PHOTO 5.2 Backhand Overhead Ceiling Shot Sequence.

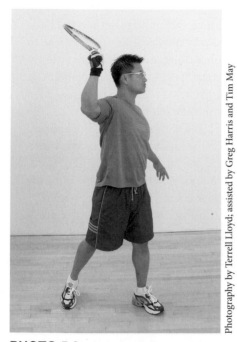

PHOTO 5.3 Laid-back Racquet for Forehand Overhead Ceiling Shot.

Photography by Terrell Lloyd; assisted by Greg Harris and Tim May

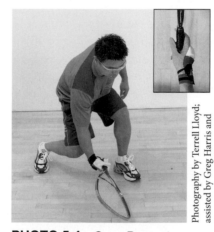

PHOTO 5.4 Open Racquet for Ceiling Shot.

Photography by Terrell Lloyd; assisted by Greg Harris and Tim May. Inset Photo by Eric Risberg

or backhand stroke. The pivot to the side wall is followed by the backswing with the wrist cocked.

As the forward swing is begun, however, the racquet head must be turned back, or "opened," toward the ceiling (see Photo 5.4). This racquet face position directs the ball toward the ceiling. Although this can be an effective shot for novice players, more advanced players usually take advantage of the low position of the ball in relation to the front wall to try to

hit an offensive return rather than a ceiling–front wall return.

To ensure the most difficult return possible, the ceiling–front wall shot should be directed to run along a side wall before it bounces into the back corner. If, in addition, the ball is directed to your opponent's backhand side, this defensive shot may result not only in a weak return but possibly no return at all. Thus, this defensive shot actually might score a point for you.

Because a ceiling–front wall shot can be hit from any part of the court, it should be practiced from all court positions. If you are standing to one side of center, you can hit the shot down the closest wall (wallpaper shot) or hit cross-court to the opposite corner.

The cross-court ceiling shot requires more power in the stroke because of the longer diagonal court distance to be covered, as well as the need for accurate placement. If the ball is not hit at a sharp angle, the rebound forward will be away from the side wall and will provide for easy stroking room. A similar problem exists with a ceiling shot hit down the line if it does not hug the wall.

Thus, although the ceiling shot is one of the easiest defensive strokes to learn, if the player does not take time to practice placement, he/she cannot achieve the true advantage of the shot. If the ceiling shot is hit well, it can be used to (1) keep the ball in play, (2) move your opponent to a back-court position, and (3) force a return that is not an offensive shot.

POINTS to REMEMBER

When the ball hits the racquet, direct the angle of the racquet head to the spot on the ceiling that you want the ball to hit.

To hit a ceiling shot from a ball below waist level, open the racquet face.

With ceiling shots hit with an overhead stroke, contact the ball just off the forward foot with an extended arm.

For the best advantage, angle ceiling shots so they rebound into a back corner, preferably to your opponent's backhand.

Lob Shot

A lob shot is not played as often as other defensive shots in competitive racquetball. This is because of the popularity of the composite/graphite racquets and pressurized balls. The lob requires finesse and placement, not the power and strength for which this equipment was designed. Therefore, players who choose a fast-moving power game often do not have the finesse necessary to hit a lob return.

A lob is used to hit a ball below head level with a technique similar to a ceiling shot. Both shots, whether hit with a forehand or a backhand stroke, require an open racquet face.

Contact with the ball should be made inside the forward foot with an extended arm. Although not much force is required to hit this ball properly, the ball should be struck with your weight shifted toward the front wall. Finish the stroke with a follow-through high over your head. This arm motion and the racquet face angle serve to lift the ball (see Photo 5.5A–E).

The lob should be returned high to the front wall, approximately six to eight feet from the ceiling. The lob shot differs from the ceiling shot in that the ball never rebounds to touch the ceiling. Rather, the ball slowly moves along an arc close to the ceiling and high over center court, falling "dead" into a back corner with little or no rebound from the back wall.

If a softer lob is hit, the ball will bounce more than once before striking the back wall. Either shot is effective, especially if hit to the opposite back corner from your opponent's position. When hit perfectly, the slow movement of this ball allows you time to reposition yourself on the court, yet forces your opponent into the disadvantage of a back-corner return (see Figure 5.2).

Similar to the ceiling shot, a lob may be hit down-the-line (along the wall) or cross-court. If the lob is hit down-the-line, it is preferable to use a backhand stroke toward the nonracquet side wall and a forehand stroke to the racquet-hand side wall for more control.

A cross-court lob may be hit with either stroke. The purpose of both shots is to place the ball in a back-court position to prevent an offensive return.

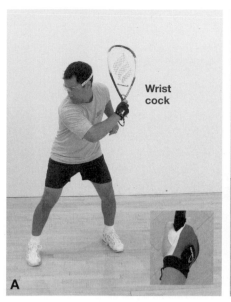

Wrist cock

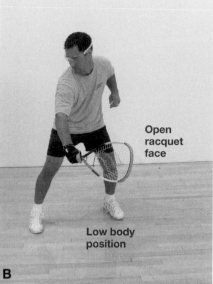

Open racquet face

Low body position

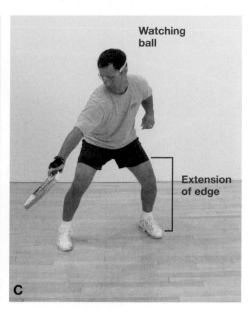

Watching ball

Extension of edge

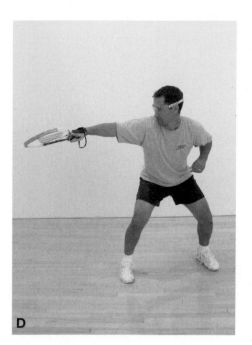

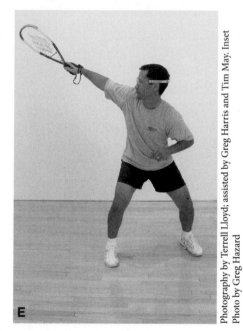

PHOTO 5.5   Backhand Lob Shot Sequence.

Photography by Terrell Lloyd; assisted by Greg Harris and Tim May. Inset Photo by Greg Hazard

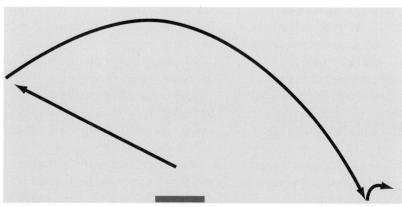

FIGURE 5.2   Proper Lob Defensive Shot.

Thus, the lob presents many of the same problems to your opponent as the ceiling shot does. The reason it is not hit more often is that it is a difficult shot to hit correctly. The ball does not rebound from the ceiling on the way to the back court. If hit too hard, the ball will merely rebound off the back wall into a center-court position (see Figure 5.3). Thus, the advantage of a back-corner placement is lost.

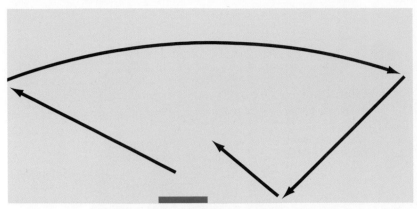

FIGURE 5.3   Lob Shot Rebounding into Center Court off Back Wall.

In addition, because the ball moves so slowly, it is easy to hit a strong return unless the lob is placed correctly. To minimize any possible rebound off the back wall, aim the lob so the ball just brushes against a side wall close to the back corner.

This "meeting" will slow the ball and deaden its fall to the floor.

For most beginners, the finesse with which this ball must be hit is hard to manage in a game situation, where quick movements are necessary.

Yet, the lob does offer an interesting variation, including changing the pace of the game, for players who can use it.

POINTS *to* REMEMBER

Pivot the hips and hit the ball with an open racquet face.

Hit the ball as hard as you think necessary, then take some force off your swing.

Finish the stroke with a follow-through, with the racquet ending up high over your shoulder.

To take some power out of your shot, aim the ball to "brush" the side wall close to the back corner.

To be more effective, lob only to a back corner.

High-Z Ball (Three-wall Shot)

Like the other defensive shots, the high-Z ball, or three-wall shot, is designed to move the opponent into a back corner. The high-Z can be hit with either an overhead stroke from a high ball or a forehand or backhand stroke on a low ball return.

To ensure proper placement of the ball, the racquet head at contact must again be angled in the direction toward which the ball should travel. This means the racquet face should be slightly open. In all other respects, the high-Z stroke resembles one of the other defensive shots. The overhead stroke is similar to the overhead ceiling shot, and the high-Z hit from a lower ball is similar to the lob.

As in other defensive shots, the high-Z must be directed to hit high off the front wall. In addition, this shot must hit close to a front wall–side wall seam (two to three feet from it). As a result, the ball, after contact with the front wall, rebounds off the nearest side wall and moves diagonally across the court to the back corner.

In essence, the movement of the ball describes a "Z" in the court. To follow this path (see Figures 5.4 and 5.5), the ball must not hit the ceiling.

Placement of the ball on the front wall is critical to the effectiveness of this shot. If hit too low, the Z ball is an easy setup for your opponent. This

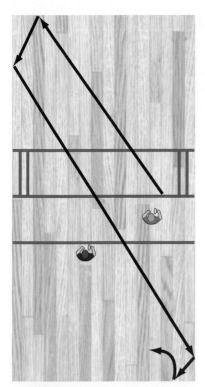

FIGURE 5.4 High-Z (Three-wall) Defensive Shot.

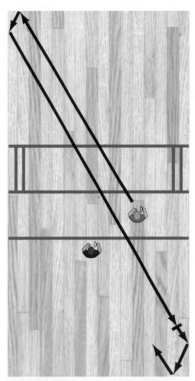

FIGURE 5.5 High-Z Defensive Shot Hitting Floor Before Back Corner.

rebounds to the floor (see Figure 5.4). Thus, the name "three"-wall is often used to identify this shot. In this situation, the ball will "run the corner" by hitting in succession the side wall, the back wall, and then the floor. The ball also may hit the floor before a second wall is touched, deadening its movement as well (see Figure 5.5).

Because the ball covers so much of the court on a Z-ball return, beginning players often do not have a powerful enough stroke to hit the shot well. It is good to practice this shot often and feel confident about hitting it before trying a Z-ball return in a game situation.

Although a Z ball may be hit from anywhere in the court, you should try it from a center-court position if your shot is weak. Stronger players will be effective with a high-Z hit even from the back court. Because of the path the ball follows, the Z is best hit to the opposite corner from your court position. Otherwise, the angle off the front wall will not be great enough to cause a rebound along the diagonal.

The Z ball or three-wall shot is effective in causing a weak return, especially if the ball "runs the corner." The back corner allows little room to place a racquet and stroke through the ball unless the timing is perfect, with a good wrist snap.

Therefore, more experienced players often hit this shot to force a bad court position and to "handcuff" the opponent as well.

is because the ball passes over a center-court position when following the diagonal. A ball hit too low will pass through the center-court area within arm's reach of your opponent. As long as the ball is hit high off the front wall, it will pass high over the center court and force your opponent into a backcourt position to return the ball.

Depending upon the strength of the hit, the Z ball may or may not hit a second side wall before touching the floor in the back corner. If hit hard, a second wall will be hit on the opposite side from the first before the ball

POINTS to REMEMBER

Hit the ball high off the front wall and close to the side wall–front wall seam.

Use a stroke similar to an overhead ceiling shot for a ball over your shoulder, and a lob return for waist-high and lower balls.

Hit the ball hard enough to "run the corner" of the back court.

Hit the high-Z to the corner opposite the side of the court in which you are positioned.

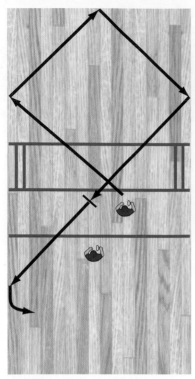

FIGURE 5.6   Around-the-Wall Ball.

Around-the-Wall Ball

The around-the-wall ball is a defensive shot that hits three walls before touching the floor. It differs from the high-Z shot in that the ball is first hit high to a side wall. The ball then rebounds to the front wall and finally to the side wall opposite from the initial hit. The closer to the front wall–side wall seam the ball is aimed, the farther back on the opposite side wall the ball will rebound.

Because the purpose of this shot, like other defensive shots, is to force the opponent into a back-court position, hitting close to a front corner is advised. If the ball strikes the first side wall too far from the front, the rebound will merely follow a path back to a center-court position (see Figure 5.6).

The stroke used to hit an around-the-wall ball is the same as for the high-Z. This shot must be practiced, however, to ensure that the proper racquet angle is used to hit the ball close to the front corner. Although not used often, the around-the-wall shot is probably most effective against a beginning player who has difficulty determining the rebound angle of the ball, or against any player to change the pace of the game.

POINTS *to* REMEMBER

Hit the around-the-wall ball with the same technique used for a high-Z ball.

For the most effective hit, angle the ball close to the front wall–side wall seam.

Use this ball against beginning players and as a change of pace.

COMMON ERRORS **HOW TO CORRECT THEM**

1. My ceiling shots never hit the ceiling.

   If the ball is hit from a position below the waist, you are not hitting with an open racquet face to lift the ball high enough to hit the ceiling. If you are using an overhead stroke, the ball is probably too far in front of you when you contact it, or your racquet head is not angled toward the ceiling to direct the ball upward.

2. My ceiling shots hit the ceiling straight over my head.

   For both waist-level and overhead shots, you have angled your racquet too much, and the racquet face is almost parallel to the ceiling. In addition, with the overhead stroke, the ball is probably contacted over your head rather than off your forward foot.

3. My lob always hits the ceiling.

   You have too much force in your hit or too much angle on the racquet head. Hit the ball softer, and aim for a point lower on the front wall.

4. My lob always hits the back wall and rebounds to center court.

   Try to angle the hit more into the back corner of the court, then limit the force with which you hit the ball. If the ball does rebound into the court, at least it will be along the wall and still will provide little stroking room.

5. My high-Z does not hit the back-wall corner but goes straight into the back wall.

   Angle your hit into the front wall closer to the front wall–side wall seam by changing the direction of the racquet head.

6. My high-Z bounces too high off the back wall and gives my opponent an easy return.

   Hit the ball lower to the front wall, or softer and with more of an open racquet face so the ball arcs into the back court.

7. My high-Z ball always rebounds off the front wall–side wall and bounces at center court, where my opponent returns it.

   Make sure that you are pivoting your hips before you stroke and that you are stepping into the ball. If you rely only on the strength of your arm to hit the ball, the force may not be great enough and the ball may not complete the diagonal of the court before touching the court floor.

CHECKPOINTS

Answers are located on page 141.

1. A ceiling–front wall shot should hit the ceiling:
   a. at the ceiling–front wall seam.
   b. two to three feet from the ceiling–front wall seam.
   c. after hitting the front wall.
   d. in the middle, halfway to the back wall.

2. The hardest court position to return a ball is:
   a. in the front court.
   b. in the middle of the service zone.
   c. just behind the short line.
   d. in a back corner close to both the back and side walls.

3. A ceiling–front wall shot can be hit:
   a. from a ball below waist level.
   b. from a ball above your head.
   c. with both a forehand and a backhand shot.
   d. all of the above.

4. If the ceiling-front wall shot is hit properly, it can be used to:
   a. keep the ball in play.
   b. move your opponent to a back-court position.
   c. force a return that is not an offensive shot.
   d. all of the above.

5. A three-wall shot:
   a. follows the path of a "V" across the court.
   b. is an offensive shot.
   c. is designed to rebound into the back court.
   d. all of the above.

6. A ceiling–front wall shot:
   a. can be hit from almost any court position.
   b. must be hit very softly to be useful.
   c. is very difficult to learn.
   d. should not be used often in the game.

7. To hit a lob shot correctly high to the front wall but not touch the ceiling :
   a. requires finesse and placement.
   b. use a technique similar to a ceiling shot.
   c. the ball should be returned.
   d. all of the above

8. What all defensive shots have in common is:
   a. they are difficult to learn
   b. they require a lot of strength
   c. they should rebound the ball into the back court
   d. you can only hit them from the front court

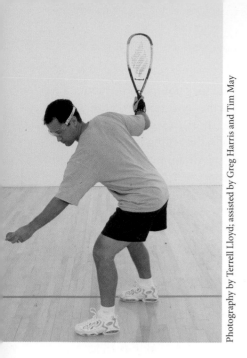

Photography by Terrell Lloyd; assisted by Greg Harris and Tim May

6

Serves in Racquetball

Serving is the most important offensive weapon in the arsenal of a beginning player. The serve can either set up a winning shot or prevent the opponent from scoring on the return of serve. The effectiveness of the serve depends on the controlled way in which it can be hit. This is the only time you can contact the ball in a position of your choosing. Thus, you can play to your strengths or your opponent's weaknesses if you can consistently serve your best shot.

There are only four basic serves. Each serve, however, can be changed to give a slightly different look by varying the power with which it is hit, its height of rebound off the front wall, or the angle of rebound into the back court. With these variations, the basic serves can become hundreds of different shots.

The wise player mixes the variations to keep the opponent guessing as to where the next ball will be served. The serve chosen should be hit only after giving thought to the opponent's strengths and skills.

Even a well-placed serve, if hit so an opponent can return it with a favorite shot, is nothing more than a nice setup. Similarly, a good player never hits a weak serve merely for the sake of variety if it is not obvious

that an equally weak return will follow.

To make the serve variations effective, your serve must not become predictable, either from the position you take in the service zone or from the technique with which you strike the ball. Ideally, all serves are hit from a similar position on the court, with a similar stroke.

Usually, the center of the service zone and a normal forehand stroke are used. In this way, it is difficult, if not impossible, for your opponent to anticipate the direction of your serve.

This means that variation in your serve must be a result of the amount of wrist snap or the position of the racquet face at the moment of contact with the ball. Either factor will affect the angle of hit or the power of the stroke.

Because you as the server are the only one who knows where the serve will be hit, you also should anticipate placement of the returned ball. Therefore, take the time before each serve to plan the best serve and also the most likely return and how best to play the ball. Ideally, if the serve is not an outright winner, at least a poor return should result, setting you up for your best offensive stroke.

For an opponent you have never seen play, a good strategy is simply

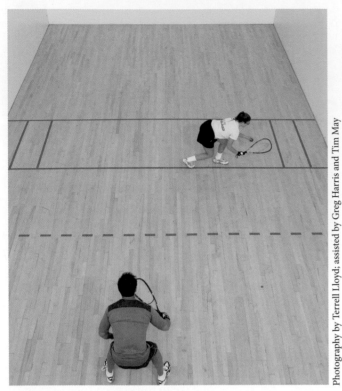

Photography by Terrell Lloyd; assisted by Greg Harris and Tim May

PHOTO 6.1   Serving position on the court.

to serve to the backhand court with your best serve. If a player has a weakness, it usually is on the backhand side. This strategy should increase the odds of your winning the point with your serve.

The serve provides the server with the offensive advantage in the game. To serve without purpose or thought to your opponent's skill gives up this advantage, and possibly the serve with it.

Legal Serves

To make a legal serve, you must hit the ball after it rebounds off the floor within the service zone. After contact with the racquet, the ball must strike the front wall before any other part of the court. But the rebounding ball from the front wall may touch one side wall before falling to the floor behind the short line.

The ball may not touch the floor in front of the short line or on the short line (short), a second side wall (three-wall), the ceiling (ceiling), or the back wall (long) before the ball makes contact with the floor. A three-wall, short, long, or ceiling serve is an illegal serve—a fault—and should not be played. A fault also is called if the server does not begin the serve with both feet in the service zone or steps out of the service zone before the ball crosses the short line after rebounding off the front wall, called a foot fault.

If a fault occurs, a second service opportunity is awarded to the server. Two faults during one service attempt result in a loss of serve (out).

A loss of service (out) also occurs if the ball is hit before it rebounds off the floor, it makes contact with the floor or any other surface before the front wall, it rebounds off the front wall and makes contact with the server or the server's racquet, the server swings but does not hit the ball, the ball hits a front wall seam, or the ball is hit illegally. If any of these actions occur, an out is called and service is lost.

A complete explanation of the rules related to serving is given in Chapter 11, page 105, as well as in the Official Rules of Racquetball in the Appendix.

Most serves are hit with a forehand stroke. The server stands as far back as possible in the service zone with the hips pivoted, facing the side wall (see Photos 6.1 and 6.2).

This provides as much service zone as possible in which to step forward when contacting the ball. Stepping out of the service zone during the serve is illegal (fault).

To begin the serve, the ball is released off the fingertips of the non-racquet hand and dropped to the floor. The hand should be extended to the front wall so the ball is dropped as far forward as possible in the service zone (see Photo 6.3).

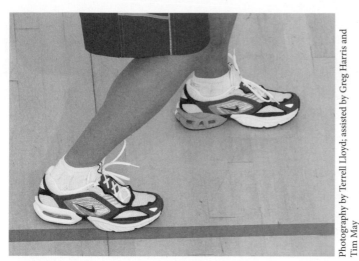

PHOTO 6.2 Foot Placement to Begin Serve.

Photography by Terrell Lloyd; assisted by Greg Harris and Tim May

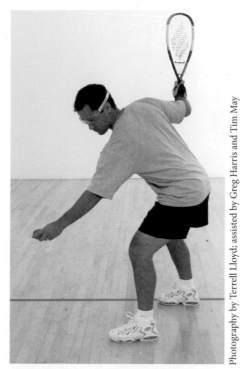

PHOTO 6.3 Ball Dop for Service.

Photography by Terrell Lloyd; assisted by Greg Harris and Tim May

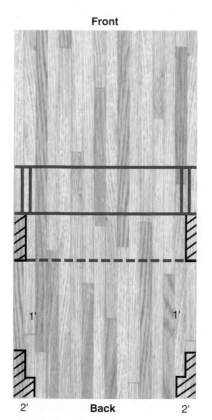

Front

Back

2'   2'

1'   1'

FIGURE 6.1 Optimal Court Areas for Served Ball to be Directed.

If the ball is not dropped close to the service line (front part of the service zone), the server will move past the ball when stepping forward to hit it. Thus, the ball will be contacted off the back foot, and much of the force of the stroke will be lost.

At the beginning of the serve, the racquet has already completed the backswing and is held perpendicular to the back wall. When the ball leaves the hand, the forward swing of the racquet begins. The angle of the racquet head and the height of the ball off the floor at contact are dependent upon the type of serve being hit. In any serve, however, it is essential to step into the stroke.

Shifting the body's weight from the back of the service zone to the foot that steps toward the service line provides additional power.

As with any other stroke, the serve is completed with a follow-through, the final position of the racquet being dependent upon the type of serve used. It is important to always hit

through the ball rather than merely punch at it. Although most serves are hit with a forehand stroke, on occasion a backhand stroke may be used.

The following four serves—the drive serve, the Z serve, the lob, and the garbage serve—are designed to follow the rules of service as well as place the opponent in a poor court position from which to hit an offensive return. As described with defensive strokes, this means serving the ball into a back corner of the court.

On all serves, it is important to keep the ball in the back corners and away from the midline of the court (see Figure 6.1).

A return from the middle of the court provides too many opportunities for offensive shots and prevents the server from holding a center-court position. Thus, the following serves should be directed wide of the midline of the court and should rebound back to a center-court position only after bouncing twice on the floor and being ruled a dead ball.

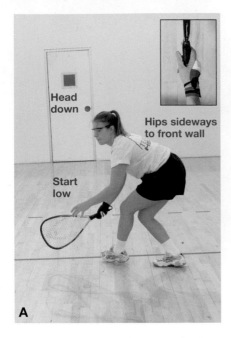

Head down

Hips sideways to front wall

Start low

A

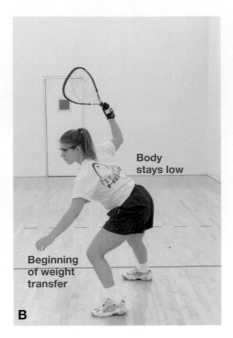

Body stays low

Beginning of weight transfer

B

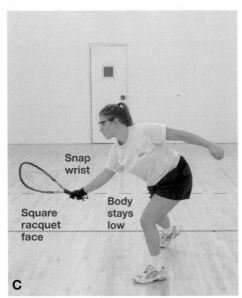

Snap wrist

Square racquet face

Body stays low

C

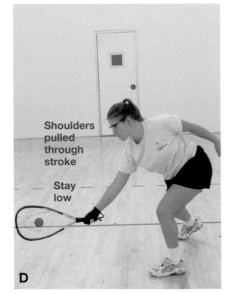

Shoulders pulled through stroke

Stay low

D

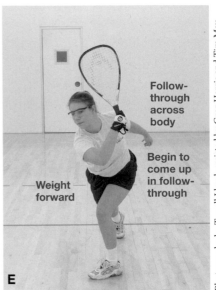

Follow-through across body

Begin to come up in follow-through

Weight forward

E

Photography by Terrell Lloyd; assisted by Greg Harris and Tim May.
Inset Photo by Eric Risberg

PHOTO 6.4   Drive Serve Sequence.

Drive Serve

A drive serve is hit with a strong forehand stroke to ensure good speed on the ball. To maximize the power in the stroke, you must begin the serve with your hips sideways to the front wall and meet the ball by stepping toward it during the forward swing. The ball should be contacted close to the floor—somewhere between the bent knee and the ankle.

The forward swing should be level to the ground and the ball met just inside the forward foot.

The follow-through should be across the body and should pull the shoulders around to finish the stroke facing the front wall. This serve resembles the kill shot in technique (see Photos 6.4A–E).

To be most effective, the drive serve must be hit low to the front wall to ensure a low ball rebounding into

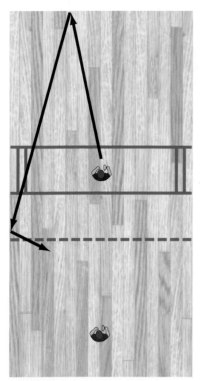

FIGURE 6.2   Short Corner Drive Serve.

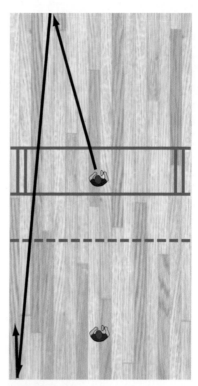

FIGURE 6.3   Drive Serve to Back Corner.

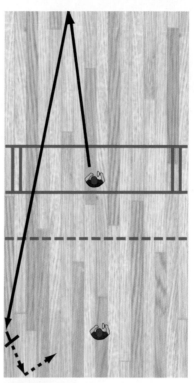

FIGURE 6.4   Drive Serve off Side Wall.

the back court. Keeping the ball low adds to the difficulty in the return.

The drive serve is not directed to any one particular area of the court. As in other serves, however, the serve should not rebound close to the midline of the back court. As illustrated in Figure 6.2, the ball can hit the side wall just past the short line (short corner drive serve). The serve can also go straight into the back corner of the court (see Figure 6.3), or hit the side wall several feet from the back wall and rebound around the back corner (see Figure 6.4).

Any of these serves will be effective as long as you vary the angle of rebound off the front wall from serve to serve and keep the ball low.

To do this, the angle of the racquet face at ball contact must change with each hit. To prevent your opponent from anticipating the position of your serve, learn to hit a drive serve to the forehand and backhand sides of the court with equal skill. The backhand side is most effective in preventing offensive returns.

Z Serve

The Z serve can be divided into two distinct serves: a high-Z serve and a low-Z serve. The high-Z serve is similar to the defensive Z shot in its movement around the court. This serve hits high on the front wall close to the front wall–side wall seam. The ball rebounds to the nearest side wall, then travels high across the diagonal of the court to the opposite back corner.

For the serve to be legal, the ball must hit the floor before touching another wall (unlike the defensive Z shot) and rebounding again.

Thus, the movement of the ball on the court resembles the letter Z.

This Z serve is hit with the same technique as the defensive Z shot.

The hips are turned to the side wall, the racquet face is open, and contact with the ball is made inside the forward foot. The stroke cannot be as strong as the defensive shot because the ball must touch the floor before striking the opposite side wall. Thus, the high-Z serve requires

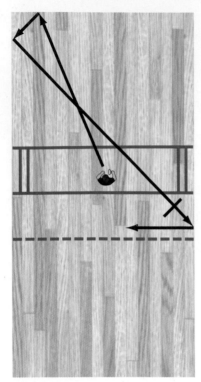

FIGURE 6.5   Low-Z Serve with Spin Hitting Past Short Line.

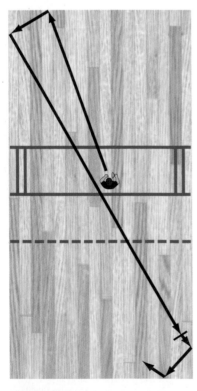

FIGURE 6.6   Low-Z Serve Directed to Back Corner of Court.

proper placement and finesse, rather than power, to be effective.

At the opposite extreme, the low-Z serve requires power to make the shot work. The low-Z serve follows the same Z path around the court, but instead of traveling above shoulder height, the ball moves through the court close to the ground. Thus, this serve is hit low to the front wall, similar to the drive serve but with more strength because the ball must travel farther (past the short line) before touching the floor.

The technique used to hit a low-Z serve is similar to that for a kill shot (see Chapter 4). The ball must be contacted inside the forward foot as the weight shifts forward. The racquet should have a level swing at contact with the ball, and the arm movement must be completed with a follow-through. Punching at the ball by stopping the racquet's motion after hitting the ball will limit the power of the swing. A good wrist snap is also essential in providing the power necessary to hit a low-Z ball.

The low Z may rebound to the floor anywhere along the side wall past the short line. If the ball is hit hard and close to the front wall–side wall seam, the ball will rebound to the floor just behind the short line and hit the side wall (see Figure 6.5). The extreme spin on the ball, because of the power of the stroke, will cause the ball to rebound perpendicular to the side wall. An opponent positioned to hit a ball served deep into a back corner will be out of place to return this serve.

If the ball is hit several feet from the front wall–side wall seam, the ball will be directed toward the back corner of the court (see Figure 6.6).

The different angles that can be used to hit the low-Z serve depend on the angle of the racquet head when the ball is contacted. The variety of angles provides another means of preventing your opponent from knowing where to set up for the return of serve.

To be most successful, the low-Z serve requires a powerful and accurate stroke. If the ball is moving too slowly, the opponent may be tempted to hit the ball as it passes through the center-court position.

For this reason, the low-Z serve is used primarily by experienced players and seldom by beginning players who have not mastered shifting their body weight and snapping the wrist to increase the power of the serve.

Beginning players usually rely on the high-Z serve. Although this serve results in a slow-moving ball, it can be especially effective if hit to the backhand of a hard-hitting opponent because of its placement into a back corner.

Lob

The lob serve is hit in a similar fashion as the lob defensive shot.

The serve may be hit cross-court or down-the-line. As in the defensive lob, the ball must be hit high to the front wall (15 feet off the floor), and the rebound should bounce the first time in the safety zone near the receiving line. The second bounce will be deep in the court near the back wall. To do this, upon the forward swing of the stroke, the racquet face must be held slightly open to the ceiling. The ball is contacted at waist level. The stroke is finished with the racquet held high over the forward shoulder (see Photos 6.5A—E). As in the defensive lob, a lob serve requires finesse rather than power.

To ensure that the ball will die in the back court, the lob serve can graze a side wall close to the back wall. This rebound will slow the movement of the ball. As a result, the serve must be directed accurately to a corner. Accuracy in placement is critical. If the ball does not "handcuff" your opponent in the back corner,

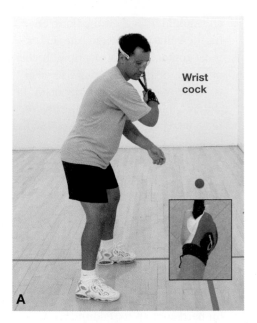

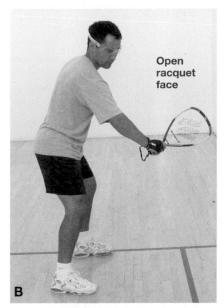

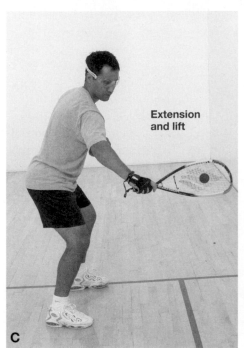

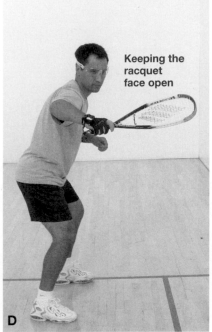

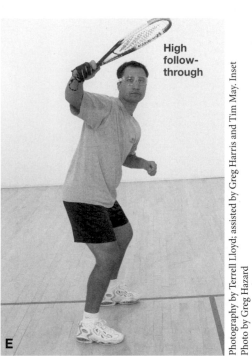

Photography by Terrell Lloyd; assisted by Greg Harris and Tim May. Inset Photo by Greg Hazard

PHOTO 6.5   Backhand Lob Serve Sequence.

this slow-moving ball will be an easy setup for an offensive return.

If this is difficult for you to do, hit the serve to the opponent's backhand.

This will provide for a margin of error in placement because it will force a weak side return.

To increase the accuracy of the lob serve to the backhand side of the court, many players change their center-court serving position and move to that side of the service zone.

In addition, they hit the ball with a backhand stroke, using an open racquet face as on the forehand side. Although there is little deception in this maneuver, the difficulty in returning a lob serve comes not in surprising the opponent as much as in placing the ball. This court position allows for better placement because the ball is not hit at an angle. Rather, the racquet is parallel to the front wall and the ball is hit straight.

The lob is a good serve to use to change the pace of the game and to slow down a fast-moving opponent who likes to return serves hard to the front wall. This is because the return of serve cannot be made until the ball either bounces or passes the plane of the receiving line. This forces a defensive return. Again, accuracy of placement is crucial to the success of this serve.

Garbage Serve

A garbage serve is hit with a forehand stroke. This serve looks much like a drive serve. The forward swing is level with the floor, and the ball is contacted inside the front foot. The force of the hit is dependent upon the speed of the swing and the snap of the wrist when the ball is contacted.

The ball should not be hit as hard as it is in a drive serve, or as softly as a lob. Yet, the follow-through should draw the racquet across the body to hit "through the ball." Although the ball should rebound wide of the midline of the court, it is not hit low to the floor or high to the ceiling. Rather, the ball rebounds into the back court at a height between the opponent's waist and shoulder level off the floor. To hit the ball to this height, the server must contact the ball at a point higher off the floor than for a drive serve or with the racquet face slightly open. In general, the movement of the ball on the court gives the impression that the ball has been mishit.

This serve may or may not be hit with enough angle to rebound off a side wall before entering the back court. If it is, the ball should just brush the side wall so the ball does not rebound back into play. In this respect, a garbage serve is similar to a lob.

If the serve is directed straight into the back corner, the ball must not be hit hard enough to rebound strongly off the back wall after hitting the floor. A strong rebound at this point will negate the value of the garbage serve. The strategy behind this serve is to force a ceiling return or to prevent your opponent from hitting a kill shot or other offensive return. This strategy is especially effective with an opponent who can hit offensive shots consistently off your best serve, placing you immediately on the defensive. Using a garbage serve should at least get you past the serve and on to other opportunities to win the point.

POINTS *to* REMEMBER

Unless a serve requires a different court position, serve from the center of the service zone with a forehand stroke so you don't signal the type of serve you will hit.

Never serve the ball down the midline of the court, where an offensive return is easy to hit.

In addition to hitting the serve wide of the middle of the court, hit the ball low unless a garbage, lob, or high-Z serve is desired.

If you don't know your opponent, serve to the backhand side of the court.

Practice hitting your serves to rebound at different angles off the front wall, using varying heights off the floor and changing the power in your stroke.

The closer to the center of the front wall the ball is hit, the farther back in the court the ball will strike a side wall. The closer to a front wall corner the ball strikes, the closer to the front wall the ball will hit the side wall.

To change the pace of the game or to force a ceiling ball return, use a lob or a high-Z serve.

COMMON ERRORS **HOW TO CORRECT THEM**

1. My lob serve hits the ceiling or the back wall.

   You are hitting the ball too hard or with too much angle toward the ceiling. Hit the ball softer and with less angle so the ball will hit lower on the front wall.

2. My drive serve rebounds off the back wall into the center court.

   Bend your knees, bringing your body closer to the floor so you can drop your racquet lower to the floor. This will allow you to contact the ball when it is closer to the floor. Hitting a lower ball into the back court will lessen the chance of a rebound off the back wall.

   In addition, angling the ball to hit a side wall before it touches the back court floor should deaden the movement of the ball into the back court and prevent a hard rebound from the back wall.

3. My Z serve hits two side walls before it hits the floor.

   Hit the ball farther from the front corner and closer to the center of the front wall so the ball will rebound to a point farther into the back court. Another correction would be to hit the ball with less stroking power while keeping the same forward swing to maintain the height of the ball's contact with the front wall.

4. My drive serve pops off the front wall and rebounds high into the back court.

   You probably are standing up as you make contact with the ball during the serve. If you do not maintain a low position to the floor throughout the forward swing, the ball will be lifted along with your body and will rebound up off the front wall. Make sure that you have followed through your serving motion before you come to a ready position to prepare for the return of serve.

5. My garbage serve hits straight into the back wall.

   You are hitting the serve too hard. Take some power off your stroke, and angle the racquet head slightly toward the ceiling upon contact with the ball.

6. My serves go straight down the center of the court.

   You are not hitting the ball with enough angle (toward a front wall corner). This can be corrected in one of two ways: (1) If you want to hit the ball to the side wall behind you, throw the ball out in front of you toward your backhand side. If you want to hit the ball toward the side wall you are facing, throw the ball slightly behind the front foot and toward your forehand side. (2) If you want to serve to the side wall behind, always throw the ball in the same place relative to your body, but concentrate on breaking your wrist upon contact with the ball. If you want to hit toward the side wall you are facing, open up your wrist (laid-back position). This technique is the best because it will disguise your service direction until making contact.

CHECKPOINTS

Answers are located on page 141.

1. A service fault is called:
   a. when the ball strikes the front wall, then a side wall.
   b. when the ball hits the back wall after hitting the floor.
   c. when the ball touches the ceiling after the front wall.
   d. when the ball is hit with an over-head stroke.

2. A lob serve can be used to:
   a. change the pace of the game.
   b. overpower your opponent.
   c. slow down a hard-hitting opponent.
   d. "handcuff" an opponent against a side wall.

3. All serves should avoid:
   a. hitting the back wall before the floor.
   b. rebounding into the middle of the court.
   c. hitting the floor before the ball passes the short line.
   d. all of the above.

4. All serves should be:
   a. hit from a similar position in the service zone.
   b. struck with a similar stroke.
   c. intended to score a point or gain an advantage by setting up a winning shot.
   d. all of the above.

5. Serves can be varied by:
   a. letting the ball bounce twice before hitting it.
   b. hitting the ceiling prior to the front wall like a defensive shot.
   c. changing the angle of the racquet head at the moment of contact with the ball.
   d. hitting two side walls before the ball touches the floor.

6. The garbage serve:
   a. looks like a Z serve.
   b. almost appears to be mishit.
   c. should always be hit with a backhand stroke.
   d. should rebound strongly off the back wall.

7. The Z serve:
   a. can be hit high or low off the front wall.
   b. should hit two walls before touching the floor to be most effective.
   c. must always be hit with power because of the distance the ball travels.
   d. should always be hit to the back corner.

8. The drive serve:
   a. should be hit high off the front wall.
   b. should only be hit to your opponent's backhand side.
   c. does not have to be directed to any one particular area of the court.
   d. cannot be varied and therefore is predictable.

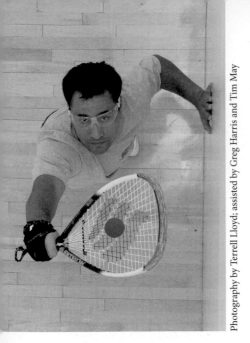

Photography by Terrell Lloyd; assisted by Greg Harris and Tim May

7

Using the Back Wall and Corners

Offensive and defensive strokes comprise the primary skills involved in the game of racquetball, but additional skills are needed to play the game to your advantage. These skills include hitting off the back wall, hitting into the back wall, and corner-shot returns.

Hitting Off the Back Wall

Up to now, this book has ignored the part of racquetball that makes it an interesting and challenging game—use of the back wall. Beginning players often learn to play racquetball by avoiding the back wall completely. As a result, they are not really playing four-wall racquetball.

This type of play puts these players at a disadvantage when facing opponents who use the whole court.

Without using the back wall as a playable surface, two problems arise: (1) any ball that gets past your position in the court is out of play with no chance for you to retrieve it, and (2) to prevent balls from getting past them, players use unorthodox strokes with unpredictable results to return the ball. Thus, when not using the

back wall, players often must resort to merely hitting the ball to keep it in play rather than directing it. We refer to this strategy as "Battleball."

When playing Battleball, the player maintains a center-court position and hits every ball within reach as hard as possible back to the middle of the front wall. The strategy is that if the ball is hit hard to the front wall, it may rebound past the opponent and score a point. Of course, this tactic may work against another Battleball player, but the experienced opponent will use the back wall skillfully to keep the ball in play. Until you feel confident enough to use the back wall, you will not be able to play more than Battleball on the racquetball court.

Patience

The key to using the back wall effectively is *patience*—the patience to let a ball intentionally go past you.

Before you can play with patience, you must develop confidence in your ability to play balls on the rebound off the back wall. Part of this confidence comes from many hours of court practice, and another part comes from understanding why the back wall is helpful.

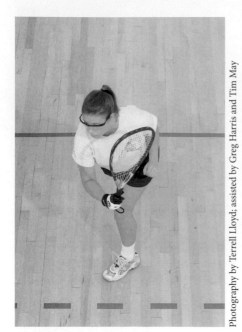

Photography by Terrell Lloyd; assisted by Greg Harris and Tim May

PHOTO 7.1   Moving for a Back Wall Return.

Back-wall Advantage

Use of the back wall provides several advantages during the game.

First, a ball that goes past you into the back court can still be hit as it rebounds off the back wall.

Second, by waiting for balls to rebound off the back wall, you can move into a better position for hitting a forehand or backhand stroke—the setup for the return. If the ball is hit before the back wall rebound, often it is above or below the ideal hitting area.

It is impossible to practice hitting balls at all positions relative to your body. Therefore, always adjusting your court position so the ball is at the same place relative to your forehand or backhand stroke will ensure a consistent hit. This means that you will be in control of the ball's movement around the court and, consequently, your opponent's court position as well.

Finally, waiting for the rebound affords you more time to see where your opponent is waiting in the court and to plan the most effective offensive return. Thus, use of the back wall adds to your ability to control movement of the ball and your opponent's court position and to potentially gain an offensive advantage.

Getting in Position

To position yourself to hit a good return off the back wall, you must never lose eye contact with the ball or turn your back to the front wall (see Photo 7.1). The most critical mistake that players make when returning balls off the back wall is turning to face the back wall when stroking the ball. As a result, a normal forehand or backhand stroke cannot be used because the ball would be hit into the side wall.

Out of desperation, then, the player facing the back wall resorts to flipping the ball over the shoulder, hitting a blind shot toward the front. This shot does not allow you to control and direct the movement of the ball—just to keep it in play.

The only way to use the back wall successfully is to pivot your hips for a forehand or backhand return and adjust your position relative to the ball's rebound by cross-stepping up or back.

The critical decision to be made when returning a ball from the back wall is whether to use a forehand or a backhand shot. This decision must be made quickly, and the pivot to the appropriate side should follow immediately.

It is easy to judge the side from which most balls should be hit. Balls that follow the diagonal of the court, however, are more difficult to play.

Usually, these balls begin in the front court close to one corner and end in the back court at the opposite corner.

Therefore, a ball that begins on your left side becomes a hit from the right side, and you must pivot to the opposite corner from where the ball rebounds in the front court. Practicing for these balls on the court is the best way to learn how to position yourself.

To properly hit any ball off the back wall, a player never can afford to stop watching the ball as it rebounds off the front wall for the back-wall hit. Follow the ball from your pivot position, moving only your eyes to keep the ball in sight.

Once the pivot to the appropriate side has been made, proper positioning for the rebound will allow you to either make or miss the shot.

It is hard to learn how to adjust your position for the ball without going into the court and practicing,

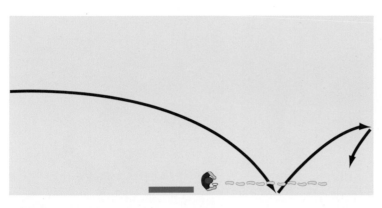

FIGURE 7.1   Move to the Back Court to Return a Ball Rebounding off Back Wall After Hitting Court Floor.

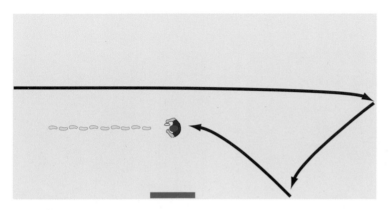

FIGURE 7.2   Move to Center Court to Return Ball Rebounding off Back Wall.

but a few general guidelines might be helpful in getting you started.

If the ball has touched the floor before it hits the back wall, you must hit it before it touches the floor again, directly off the back-wall rebound. Because it has touched the floor, the ball's bounce is deadened and will not rebound far off the back wall (see Figure 7.1). Thus, you will have to move close to the back wall to hit the ball. If the ball hits the back wall without touching the floor, you should wait for the ball to hit the floor before making contact with it. But be prepared to move forward in the court, because the ball will rebound

sharply off the wall and run toward the front-court area (see Figure 7.2). In either case, you need to position yourself so that, at the point of contact, the ball will be hit inside the forward foot with the proper forehand or backhand stroking motion (see Photo 7.2A–E).

A more difficult shot to return is the back-wall rebound of a lob or ceiling shot that just grazes the back wall, dies, and falls to the floor. With either shot, the ball has touched the floor already. Therefore, the ball must be hit immediately after contact with the back wall. The only way to hit this type of rebound successfully is with a sharp wrist snap on the racquet. Station the racquet between the path of the ball and the wall (see Photo 7.3). As the ball passes the face of the racquet, flip the racquet forward with a sharp wrist motion.

The best return on this ball is a defensive shot directed toward the top of the front wall. This way, if the shot is weak, the ball still will make contact somewhere on the front wall surface. In addition, a defensive return will give you time to reposition yourself on the court.

If, during a game, you are not able to return the ball off the back wall, you may have to hit the ball as it is falling toward you, before it strikes the back wall. In this case, the best shot to use is an overhead ceiling shot (see Chapter 5). With this return, you will keep the ball in play and have an opportunity to win the rally later.

Never jump to hit these balls. All balls eventually will fall to within arm's reach. If the ball hits so high off the back wall that it can't be hit with an outstretched arm, wait for the rebound. Jumping only adds another factor to control when trying to hit the ball perfectly. Jumping for the ball is a sign of impatience.

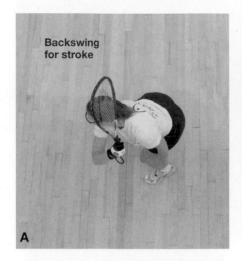

Backswing for stroke

A

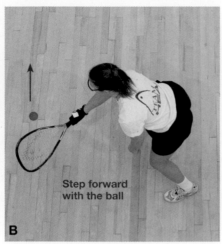

Step forward with the ball

B

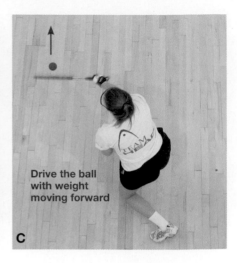

Drive the ball with weight moving forward

C

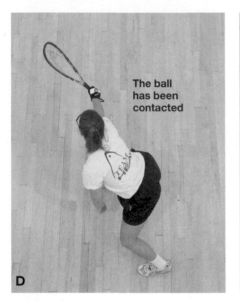

The ball has been contacted

D

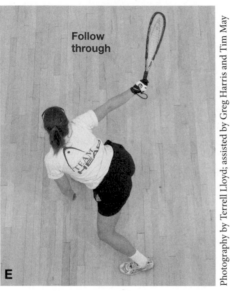

Follow through

E

PHOTO 7.2   Backhand Return off Back Wall.

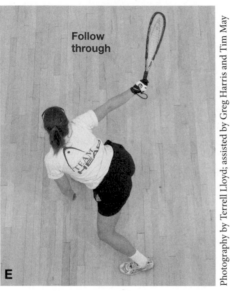

PHOTO 7.3   Placing Racquet Close to Wall to Hit Ball.

POINTS to REMEMBER

Watch the ball at all times.

To hit a ball off the back wall, pivot 90 degrees to the side from which the shot is to be taken, and cross-step forward or backward to a court position where the ball will rebound.

If the ball touches the floor before it hits the back wall, the rebound will drop close to the back wall.

If the ball hits the back wall before it touches the floor, the ball will rebound into a mid- to center-court position.

Return balls that rebound strongly off the back wall with a defensive or an offensive shot using either a backhand or a forehand stroke.

Return a ball that grazes the back wall by emphasizing the wrist snap and placing the racquet along the wall, hitting a defensive return as the ball falls past the face of the racquet.

Hitting into the Back Wall

Rather than using the back wall properly, a temptation for a beginning player is to hit the ball into the back wall with the hope that it will rebound the length of the court to the front wall. This type of hit is more likely to happen if the player turns completely around to face the back wall when playing the rebound.

For some players, hitting into the back wall becomes a favorite shot. Unfortunately, the more you rely on this shot, the weaker your game will be.

First, it is impossible to hit an offensive shot off an into-the-back wall hit. Second, even defensive shots are unreliable from this return because you are facing away from the front wall, making it almost impossible to aim the ball. Finally, with the distance the ball must travel (more than the full length of the court), the ball becomes a slow-moving, easy target for your opponent to return. Hitting the ball into the back wall, then, should be used only as a last resort when there is no other way to keep the ball in play.

The only two occasions in which this situation is likely to occur (short of your moving lazily to a good court position) are (1) off a passing shot that beats you into the back court, and (2) a ball that falls so close to the back wall from a ceiling, lob, or served ball that you cannot place your racquet between it and the wall to stroke it forward.

If you must use a back-wall return, be sure to contact the ball with an upward scooping motion to angle the rebound above your head and high toward the front wall. The ball must be hit hard.

Never hit the ball into the back wall from a mid- or center-court position. Not only is this bad strategy, but your opponent may be in the back court and, consequently, in the path of the ball. Standing 10–15 feet away from a hit ball gives your opponent little time to duck. Many serious injuries have resulted from this type of play.

The player who wants to win at racquetball cannot afford to rely on such an ineffective and dangerous shot. To avoid placing yourself in the position of hitting the ball into the back wall: (1) never turn 180 degrees to face the back wall to return a ball, and (2) move quickly to meet the ball in the court rather than being caught out of position with no other shot available.

POINTS to REMEMBER

Hit into the back wall rarely. This is a desperation shot and provides little advantage to the player except to keep the ball in play.

Never hit into the back wall from a center- or midcourt position.

When returning the ball to the back wall, use a scooping stroke to lift the ball over your head and past your face.

Hit the ball hard, as it must travel more than the length of the court.

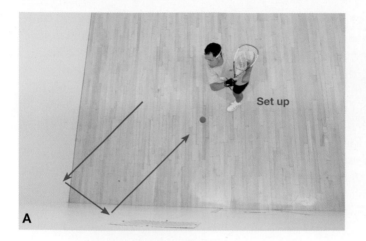

Set up

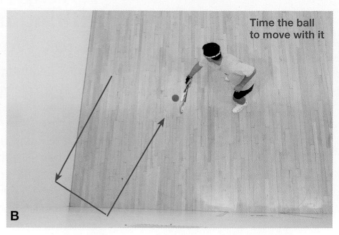

Time the ball
to move with it

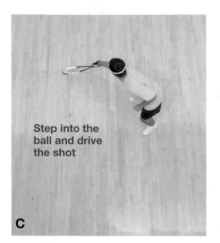

Step into the
ball and drive
the shot

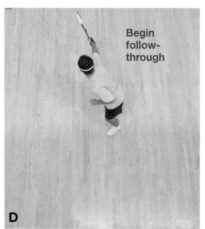

Begin
follow-
through

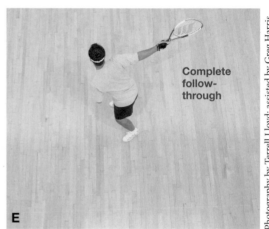

Complete
follow-
through

Photography by Terrell Lloyd; assisted by Greg Harris and Tim May

PHOTO 7.4   Hitting Out of Corner Sequence.

Corner Shots

Another important return to learn is hitting a ball that rebounds to a back corner. For most players, the corner shot return is the most difficult play in the game. To contact a corner ball, you must contend with the back and side walls simultaneously.

Without any room to stroke the ball, an effective offensive shot is eliminated and you can hope only for a good defensive return.

To play a corner shot, it is important to pivot immediately toward the corner from which the ball will rebound while keeping the ball in view. The success of this return depends upon your ability to position yourself properly in relation to the ball's movement. Anticipate the ball's rebound, and maintain a court position behind the forward bounce.

From this position you still can step into the ball to make contact. If the ball does not rebound with enough force to allow you to hit the ball with a forward swing, the power in the hit must come primarily from the wrist snap (see Photo 7.4A–E).

The last option to keep the ball in play is to hit the ball into the back wall with enough strength to have it rebound to the front wall. This strategy has been discussed previously.

The key to a successful corner shot return is having the patience to wait for the ball to rebound off the back wall. Most beginners are not patient enough to wait, and they swing wildly as the ball comes within reach. Another common mistake is to use a wide, sweeping swing with an extended arm, using the shoulder to supply the force behind the stroke. This big arm swing is dangerous, and there is no room for this type of tennis stroke in the corner of the court.

Contact with a ball in the corner that has little rebound off the back wall should be made with an open racquet face. This will direct the ball toward the ceiling and give you more margin for error. If the ball rebounds away from the back wall, any forehand or backhand return can be used. Most players choose a defensive return because of their back-court position. Therefore, the return of a corner ball should be considered successful if you hit a good defensive shot.

POINTS *to* REMEMBER

For all corner shots, position yourself behind the rebound so you can step into the ball to return it.

Avoid using a big arm swing, especially if the ball is rebounding tightly into the corner; instead, rely on a wrist snap.

If the ball does not rebound strongly out of the corner, hit a defensive ceiling shot rather than try for an offensive return.

Return a ball that rebounds hard off the corner with any type of shot.

COMMON ERRORS HOW TO CORRECT THEM

1. When I try to return a ball from a back corner, my racquet always hits a side wall.

   You are using a large arm swing to hit the ball rather than relying on the wrist snap. Place the racquet along the anticipated path of the ball, and contact the ball when it moves past the racquet face, using a sharp wrist snap.

2. When I hit a rebound off the back wall, my return always hits a side wall.

   Check to see if you are turning your hips to face the back wall rather than making only a pivot toward the side wall. This body position will cause you to hit the ball into a side wall rather than forward.

   When hitting the ball, the racquet face also could be directed at a side wall if you are contacting the ball either off your back foot or too far in front of your forward foot. Try to reposition yourself when hitting a back-wall shot so you make contact with the ball in proper position relative to your body for the stroke you are using.

CHECKPOINTS

Answers are located on page 141.

1. Using the back wall allows you to:
   a. return balls that go past you in the court.
   b. move to a better position to return a ball.
   c. note your opponent's position and hit where he/she is not.
   d. all of the above.

2. To be in a good position to hit a ball off the back wall, you should:
   a. never lose eye contact with the ball.
   b. never turn your back to the front wall when contacting the back-wall rebound.
   c. decide quickly if you will use a forehand or a backhand stroke.
   d. all of the above.

3. Beside offensive and defensive strokes, you need to develop the ability to:
   a. hit balls rebounding off the back wall.
   b. hit balls to the back wall to rebound to the front wall.
   c. hit balls rebounding off corners.
   d. all of the above.

4. Battleball is:
   a. an extremely offensive and aggressive form of racquetball utilizing the back wall.
   b. hitting the ball hard to keep it in play without a sense of strategy.
   c. useful against a player more skilled and experienced than you.
   d. none of the above.

5. Changing your court position during play is important because:
   a. you can ensure the ball is at the same place relative to your forehand or backhand stroke when returning the ball.
   b. you can use the game to enhance your aerobic condition.
   c. you can effectively block the view of your opponent to the ball.
   d. you can confuse you opponent with what type of stroke you are going to use.

6. For a beginning player, the best return of a ball that has hit the floor, grazes the back wall, and is dropping back to the floor is to:
   a. wait until the ball hits the floor, then hit a kill shot.
   b. hit a defensive shot directed toward the top of the front wall.
   c. jump and try to reach the ball before it hits the back wall.
   d. any of the above.

7. Hitting the ball into the back wall:
   a. strengthens your game by adding variety.
   b. allows you to hit an offensive shot.
   c. should only be used as a last resort.
   d. is good to hit from anywhere on the court.

8. A ball falling into the corner:
   a. is the most difficult to learn to play.
   b. usually cannot be returned with an offensive shot.
   c. requires patience to wait for the ball to rebound off the back wall.
   d. all of the above.

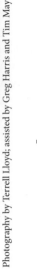

Photography by Terrell Lloyd; assisted by Greg Harris and Tim May

Putting the Strokes Together: Non-Thinking Strategy

As a beginning player on the court, your strategy is limited by your skill level. When you become more proficient with a variety of shots and feel confident enough to use them in a game situation, your strategy will change accordingly.

With limited playing skills, success on the court is obtained most easily using a defensive strategy and maintaining control of the center court. This means that your objective during each rally is to keep the ball in play with defensive shots in order to keep your opponent out of the center court and ideally, force him or her to return your shot from the back court. You can win points with this strategy, not because you make an outstanding offensive shot, but instead, because your opponent makes errors in his or her return.

At the beginning level, unforced errors account for more than half of the points scored. Therefore, if you can keep the ball in play with defensive shots, the odds are on your side that your opponent will lose the rally. This may not be as satisfying as hitting a winning shot, but it is more productive in the end. This is called the non-thinking strategy, because few decisions are made during play. The only decision you must

make is *which* defensive shot to hit and where to hit it to minimize your opponent's ability to hit an offensive return.

Why are defensive shots a good choice for a beginning player? This answer is simply because these shots are easiest to learn and consistently hit correctly.

Defensive shots can be hit hard or soft from anywhere on the court, and there is more room for error in their placement while still being strategically effective. To play a defensive game successfully, several points should be remembered:

1. Concentrate and watch the ball.
2. Serve your best.
3. Keep a center-court position.
4. Move to the ball.
5. Plan your return serve.

Concentrate and Watch the Ball

To follow any strategy when playing racquetball, you must *concentrate* on the game and *watch the ball* (see Photo 8.1). Leave any mental distractions outside the court to improve your concentration on the game, for both the players' safety and the fun of the game. A player who is distracted by other thoughts

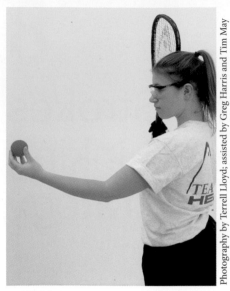

PHOTO 8.1   Concentrating and Watching the Ball.

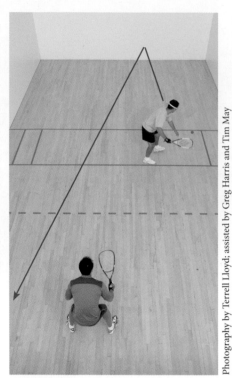

PHOTO 8.2   Serving to Back Corner.

may end up at the painful end of a well-placed stroke or, at the very least, missing easy-to-hit shots.

Concentrating on the game requires that you watch the ball at all times. This is true regardless of whether it is your turn to hit the ball. The ball moves around the court so fast, with the potential to change directions quickly, that losing eye contact with the ball usually results in an inability to properly set up for the stroke in time. Therefore, your return may result in loss of a point simply because of your poor court position.

Serve Your Best

Even though you are following a defensive strategy, you can and should use your serve to its offensive advantage. This means *serve your best.* "Best" can be defined in two ways: (1) the serve you hit well with predictable results, or (2) the serve

that might not be hit skillfully but attacks the opponent's weakness in service return.

How would you choose between these two options? Usually the choice is automatic. If a certain type of serve (such as a lob to the backhand side) always gains a point for you through a faulty return, use it. If your opponent has no consistent weakness with one type of serve, use the serve in which you are most skilled—one that you place properly and hit with authority.

Unfortunately, when you are playing a new opponent, it will take time and possibly some lost serves before you can discover a player's weakness or which serve is working best for you that day. In this case, a good strategy is to serve to the opponent's backhand. For most beginning players, the backhand suffers from a lack of practice because the player hits forehand strokes with more success. Therefore, backhand strokes are not controlled as skillfully.

In addition to hitting toward the backhand side, a serve can be more effective if the ball is hit so the rebound lands close to a side wall in a back corner (see Photo 8.2). This court position makes the serve more difficult to return with an offensive stroke. Also, your opponent must move from the middle of the court to return the ball. Consequently, this court position is open for you to occupy.

If you still are confused as to how to serve the ball, use your own experience as a guide. The serve that is most difficult for you to return will be the most difficult for your opponent as well—assuming that both of you are at similar skill levels. Your service strategy does not suggest that a serve is successful only if it is an **ace**. Rather, the serve is useful if a weak return (a ball that is neither an offensive nor a good defensive shot) follows. This type of return sets you up for an easy offensive shot to the front wall and a point.

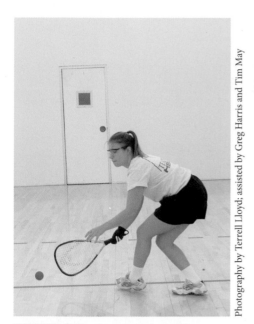

PHOTO 8.3   Service Position in Service Zone.

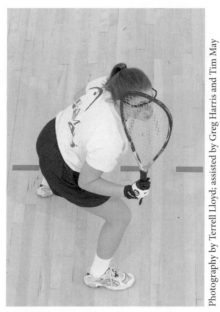

PHOTO 8.4   Center-court Position, Safely Watching the Ball.

Photography by Terrell Lloyd; assisted by Greg Harris and Tim May

Keep a Center-court Position

In a game involving beginning players, balls often pass through the center court after rebounding off the front wall. This is because the novice player returns most balls to the center of the front wall. Therefore, standing one to three feet behind the short line and an equal distance from either side wall will give you the best position to reach most balls. A center-court position is suggested only because more balls travel through this area than any other part of the court, and also because from here the player can reach balls that rebound short or long or run along either wall.

How do you gain and maintain this strategic center-court position?

If you are serving, the problem is solved easily. When playing singles, the server usually serves from a position close to the center of the service zone (see Photo 8.3). This position is taken for two reasons: (1) If all serves are hit from the same place in the service zone, there is little chance of the server's court position giving away the type of serve that is going to be hit, and (2) This position allows easy access to the strategic playing position in center court.

As soon as the server is allowed to leave the service zone, this player should back up into the center court. Because of the server's proximity to center court, a few quick steps will do the job. Unfortunately, beginning players often choose to turn, face the back wall (and the receiver who is hitting the ball), and move to a center-court position while watching the serve. This is dangerous because it exposes the server to a direct "in-the-face" return off the receiver's racquet. Also, a quick return of serve may find the server's back to the front wall as the ball rebounds.

Backing up to center court while using peripheral vision to follow the ball (see Photo 8.4) is the safest and the most effective tactic. Maintaining this court position after the serve is merely a matter of keeping your opponent out of it. To do this, place your shots consistently so the rebound off the front wall is wide of the middle of the court and deep into a back-court position. A ceiling, lob, or high-Z ball are all effective in placing the ball deep into a back-court corner.

To return these shots, your opponent must follow the ball to the back court, leaving the center-court position open for you to occupy. As long as you hit your returns in this manner, the center court will always be open.

One precaution that beginners must be aware of is to avoid hitting the ball hard enough to allow it to rebound off the back wall and into the center court. Because the player hitting the ball cannot be impeded by the opponent, a rebound of this type would force you to move out of a center-court position.

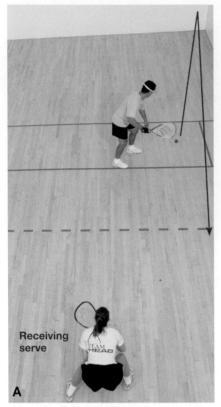
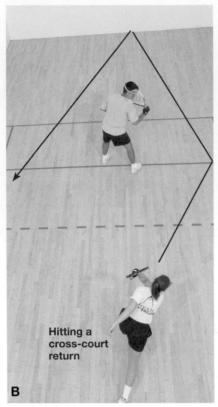
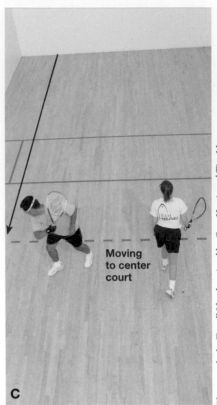

Receiving serve

A

Hitting a cross-court return

B

Moving to center court

C

Photography by Terrell Lloyd; assisted by Greg Harris and Tim May

PHOTO 8.5   Moving the Server Out of a Center-court Position.

Similarly, if you are receiving the serve, the center court will become open if you hit a defensive stroke (such as the ceiling, lob, or high-Z) along a side wall into a back corner or even a cross-court return as the server chases your return (see Photo 8.5A–C). Therefore, you should be ready to move to the center-court position once your opponent has vacated this area. The usual movement on a racquetball court consists of a constant shifting of position in and out of the center court.

The non-thinking strategy suggests returning to the center-court position after each shot as quickly as possible, or maintaining this position until moving for a ball forces you out. At the same time, you should continue to hit defensive shots away from the midline of the court to keep your opponent out of this strategic court area.

Move to the Ball

The reason you can move your opponent out of a center-court position is simply that this player must leave center court to *play the ball*.

Unfortunately, many beginning players are content to hit the ball if it is within arm's reach, regardless of where the ball is in relation to their body. This means using unorthodox strokes, few of which a player has practiced. Returns hit in this way will only rebound the ball to the front wall rather than place it. This tactic keeps the ball in play but provides neither an offensive nor a defensive advantage.

You have practiced hitting forehand and backhand shots. Why not use them? The keys to success in racquetball are knowing where to hit the ball to keep your opponent at a disadvantage and also being able to do it. Using tried and true strokes will

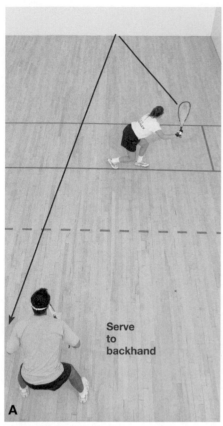

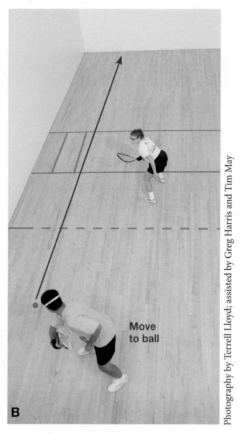

Serve to backhand

Move to ball

Photography by Terrell Lloyd; assisted by Greg Harris and Tim May

PHOTO 8.6   Moving Directly to the Ball.

stroke and generating more power in the swing, and (3) jumping is another factor that must be controlled to hit a good return.

Therefore, jumping is neither necessary nor practical as a means of moving to the ball. This is one situation in which you must wait for the ball to come to you.

Finally, when adjusting your court position to move to the ball for the best hit, you have to move to where the ball will be rather than to chase the ball around the court. Always take the shortest and most direct path to the ball's rebound (see Photo 8.6A–B). If you find this hard to do, spend some time in a court alone, hitting the ball at various angles into the front wall, and watch the ball's movement. Beginning players who have not played a court game before must learn the rebound angles and movement of the ball through experience.

produce better game results than a contrived, over-the-shoulder punch.

To hit the ball with the same stroke requires that you move to a court position where you can make the best contact with the ball. Usually this strategy involves playing balls off the back wall to allow the ball to drop from shoulder height as it moves through the court to a lower position off the back-wall rebound.

Low balls can be hit with the same forehand and backhand strokes by bending your knees and dropping your waist closer to the floor. The stroking technique remains the same.

Instead of waiting for the ball to drop from an overhead position to within arm's reach, many beginning players jump to reach the ball. Jumping is never advised as a means of getting to the ball for three reasons: (1) all balls eventually will fall to the floor and could be hit from waist level, (2) jumping for the ball prevents you from stepping into the

Plan Your Return of Serve

As a beginning player, you have to try to create an advantage in every part of the game. This includes return of serve. After a few points are played, you should be able to anticipate, or at least have an "educated guess" where and how your opponent will serve the ball. This educated guess could be a result of your opponent's position in the service zone, previous serves, or your position in the back court.

You are the observer in the first two situations. The last is dependent upon how you choose to play the serve. Taking a position in the back court that places you closer to one side wall than the other can subtly encourage your opponent to serve to the open side. This might be to your advantage if you have difficulty returning a particular serve to either your forehand or backhand. Overplaying this side of the court to discourage a serve to this area of the court actually may result in a serve that is easier for you to return. But you must be prepared to move to cover this area quickly if your strategy works!

If you stay in the center of the back court, you should at least make sure that you can look past the server to the front wall. A ball that strikes the front wall just to the right of the server usually will rebound to the back right corner of the court. A ball striking the front wall just to the left of the server will rebound into the back left corner.

Seeing where the ball hits the front wall will give you a split-second jump on the ball and hopefully will allow you to position yourself for a strong return.

If your opponent is standing in the center of the service area or off to one side and hits the ball close to a front-wall corner, the ball will rebound into the opposite back corner (right front, left back *or* left front, right back). Being aware of where the ball strikes the front wall allows you to move quickly to return the ball so you can be set to return it rather than just react to a bouncing serve.

In any case, before the serve is hit, you should plan how you are going to return the serve. This decision should be made for a serve to either your forehand or backhand and for a ball that must be hit above or below your waist. Following the non-thinking defensive strategy, a defensive return would tend to be your first choice. This is especially true if you strike the ball above your waist.

If the ball drops below your waist before you return the serve, you may decide that a passing shot is a better choice. This will be a better choice if your opponent steps back from the serve area, exposing an open court along one side wall.

A down-the-wall pass or cross-court pass to this open court can be effective at moving the opponent away from the center court position and even may win back the serve.

Once you have made a decision prior to the serve, don't waver. Any hesitation actually may cause you to make a poor return of serve or miss the return altogether. Winning or losing a point in racquetball often depends upon a few inches or a millisecond of time. Commit to how you are going to return the serve and then don't second-guess yourself; just execute it. Use your previous experience on the court to make these decisions. Remember—this is the non-thinking strategy!

At the beginning level, a kill shot on the return of serve, especially from the back court, is not one of the suggested options. A kill shot from this area of the court is a low-percentage shot, except for skilled players. Beginners typically succeed in this type of return of serve no more than 10 percent of the time. That means you are giving away nine points for each change of serve you might win. You should not attempt such a low-percentage shot in a game until you have more successes than failures.

Planning your return of serve is an effective means of preparing for the serve and taking away the advantage the serve often gives the server. Be confident in your plan and follow it. If after a while you find that your plan is not working as well as you need in order to win the game, change your plan. Don't stop planning.

Play the Defensive Game

In summary, playing the defensive game does not mean that the beginning player should never hit an offensive shot. Rather, this strategy tries to simplify the game by minimizing the options available to the player. To some extent, these options already are minimized by the skill of the player and the type of shot available. If an offensive shot can be made successfully, by all means use it to end the rally. The beginning player, however, usually must concentrate on merely staying in the game and keeping the ball in play, especially with a more experienced opponent. The defensive game is designed to do this.

In general, the defensive game relies only on your ability to hit a defensive shot and keep your opponent away from the offensive center-court position. This means consistently hitting high lobs, high-Z balls, or three-wall shots to a back corner while maintaining the center-court position yourself. In this type of game, *you do not win the game as much as the opponent loses it.* Regardless, you are still the victor. This is a non-thinking strategy because your return to the front wall is predetermined before the ball leaves your racquet: a defensive shot to the opponent's backhand corner.

The other part of the non-thinking strategy is your court position. Except for the time when you are moving to hit the ball, always station yourself in the offensive center-court position. This means that as soon as the ball leaves your racquet and you can move without interfering with your opponent, return (if necessary) to the center-court position.

Too often, a beginning player hits the ball and remains stationary, waiting to see where the opponent will hit the ball. If you are positioned on one side of the court or in the front or back court, you are giving away part of the court. A ball hit to the opposite side, short or long, would be almost impossible to return. Therefore, hit the ball and *move*. Where? To the center court.

This strategy is practical not just for the beginner but also for any player who is facing a stronger, quicker, and perhaps more skilled opponent. The defensive game takes away the opponent's offensive opportunities and slows the tempo of the game. If you are not able to move fast enough to position yourself for good returns, hitting a defensive return will help to slow the ball's movement and provide more time to get in position for the next shot.

Women can find a defensive game especially effective against men. Usually, men are stronger and faster and hit the ball with more power. Forcing the man to always return off slower-moving defensive shots will minimize this advantage.

In addition, the defensive shot will give you some breathing room—time to reposition yourself in the center court and catch your breath.

POINTS to REMEMBER

Begin on the offensive with your best serve, or at least with a serve that will prevent your opponent from hitting an offensive return.

After the serve, move to the center-court position and return to it after each hit.

Hit defensive shots on most of your returns, and preferably to the opponent's weak side (usually backhand).

Realize that defensive shots can slow the game and help to maintain the playing tempo at a speed at which you can compete successfully.

Use offensive shots only if they are sure winners. Otherwise, you are giving away a point.

Plan your return of serve.

CHECKPOINTS

Answers are located on page 141.

1. After hitting a return, the beginning player should:
   a. return to the center court.
   b. wait until the opponent returns the ball and move quickly to that position.
   c. move to the front court to take away a ball hit softly to the front wall.
   d. move to the back court to await a defensive return.

2. The "non-thinking" defensive strategy is good for the player who is:
   a. just beginning to play racquetball.
   b. playing a more experienced opponent.
   c. playing a stronger opponent who hits harder and moves faster.
   d. all of the above.

3. A defensive shot is a good choice for a beginning player because:
   a. these shots are easiest to learn.
   b. these shots should always be hit with power.
   c. these shots force you to stay in the back court so you can always see the full court in front of you.
   d. you never have to play the back wall (e.g., hit a ball off the back wall).

4. The best serve to hit is one that:
   a. is always to the backhand side of your opponent.
   b. rebounds to the center of the court.
   c. hits the ceiling before landing in the back court.
   d. one that challenges your opponent's weakness.

5. Maintaining a center-court position is advantageous because:
   a. most balls pass through the center court.
   b. a player can reach balls that rebound close to the front wall.
   c. a player can return balls rebounding to either side of the court.
   d. all of the above.

6. After serving, the player should:
   a. turn to the back wall to see how the opponent is returning the ball.
   b. step to a side wall to avoid being hit by a return shot.
   c. run forward to protect against a soft return to the front wall.
   d. back up to the center court and prepare to hit the opponent's return.

7. The non-thinking strategy is based on:
   a. a power game that attacks the opponent's weaknesses.
   b. court position and defensive shots.
   c. serving an "ace" each time so you never have to rally.

   d. returning the ball down the center of the court as often as possible to make it easy to get to.

8. To achieve the best stroke on the ball:
   a. jump to meet the ball, adding power to your stroke.
   b. hit the ball before it reaches the back wall regardless of its height off the floor.
   c. move to a court position that allows you to hit the ball at waist level and step into the ball if possible.
   d. stand as straight as possible to use your body as a lever.

9. Planning your return of serve requires you to:
   a. take a position in the back court that protects a weak side return.
   b. change the racquet grip before the serve is made.
   c. always try to hit an offensive shot such as a kill shot.
   d. none of the above.

10. A defensive game is effective:
    a. against a stronger, quicker, and more skilled opponent.
    b. in keeping your opponent away from the offensive center-court position.
    c. in keeping you in the game until your opponent makes a mistake.
    d. all of the above.

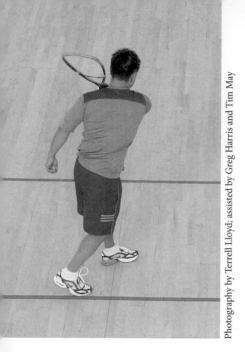

Putting the Strokes Together: Thinking Strategy

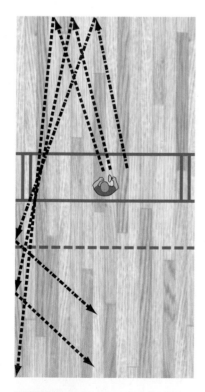

FIGURE 9.1 Different Angles of Serve and Rebound Depth.

As a player's skills improve, the non-thinking strategy of the defensive game becomes ineffective. When a player is able to add offensive strokes to his or her game with a predictable outcome, he or she must use a thinking strategy.

The strategy in this type of game involves keeping the opponent out of an offensive court position and also takes advantage of the opponent's weaknesses in skill or court position through ball placement and shot selection.

During this game, shots are varied but purposeful. The thinking strategy calls for the player to use a variety of defensive and offensive shots. Thus, points are won rather than lost, and the style of play is more aggressive. How successful a thinking/offensive strategy can be depends upon the player's skill level.

How to Choose the Right Serve

Minimally, the "right" serve is one in which an offensive shot is not returned. Ideally, the right serve results in no return to the front wall or in such a weak return that the server can hit a winning shot immediately.

Which serve will be most effective in achieving these goals will vary from opponent to opponent.

It is always a good strategy to begin by hitting your best serve to your opponent's backhand. Even if a backhand serve is anticipated, the skill of your serve should score a point. Relying continually on this serve, however, will give your opponent an opportunity to practice returning it! Variety in your serves will be the ultimate key to success at this level of play.

How can you add variety to the serve? Changing the speed of the serve, the height to the front wall, the rebound angle to the back court, or the depth to which the ball is hit in the court (see Figure 9.1) will all give your serve a new look.

The same basic serve can be hit to either side, short or long, high or low, hard or slow. In general, low, hard-hit serves (such as the drive and the low-Z) are more effective in forcing a poor return; however, this type of serve is more difficult to control. High, softer serves (such as the lob, high-Z, and garbage serve) are not as difficult to hit and, because of their placement, typically result in a ceiling shot return rather than an offensive shot.

Choosing the most effective serve for the game situation varies

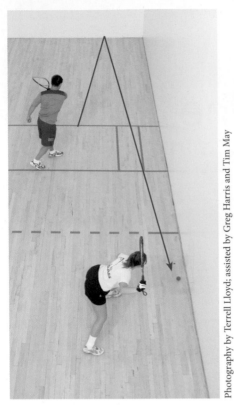

Photography by Terrell Lloyd; assisted by Greg Harris and Tim May

PHOTO 9.1   Short-drive Serve to Forehand Side, Wide of Center and Close to Side Wall.

from service to service and depends on how well you are playing. If the strengths of your game outnumber the strengths of your opponent, you can play any serve knowing that your skill should win the point. If the opponent's strengths outnumber yours, you need to play to a weakness and serve for a defensive return.

Continue to keep your opponent on the defensive until an offensive opportunity opens for you. The type of serve you choose will set the tone for your game strategy: attack and try to outgun your opponent, or play a more conservative game that keeps the opponent off the offensive.

You also may serve effectively to your opponent's forehand. Many players practice serving only to the backhand side. Serving only to this side of the court will take away some of the variety in your serve and allow your opponent to anticipate where the ball will be directed.

A serve to the forehand side can be effective if it is hit properly, is wide of center, and is close to the side wall (see Photo 9.1). If this is your opponent's strong stroke, do not serve a hard-hit ball to the forehand court. Rather, use a lob or a high-Z serve to force a defensive return.

If your opponent does not have a strong forehand shot, a low-drive serve usually will force a down-the-line return on the same side of the court. If you anticipate this return and position yourself a step closer to the side wall, your second shot of the rally can be a winner. A serve also can be effective if the return of that serve sets you up for an offensive shot, regardless of how well the return of serve is hit.

Another strategy suggests that when you are tired, you should hit your hardest serves. Assuming that you are not the player in worse shape, your feeling of fatigue undoubtedly will be matched by your opponent.

The harder the serve, the faster it must be reacted to. A tired player reacts slower or returns the ball with less power than a fresh opponent does. Take advantage of your ability to control the tempo of the game by serving hard and keeping up the pressure. This would be an excellent time to hit a short-drive serve if your opponent is playing deep in the back court.

With the serve, you control the game. It is the only time during play when you determine where the ball will be when you hit it. Use this advantage to set the tempo of the game, emphasize your strong skills, and force your opponent to rely on his or her weaknesses. At the very least, if you do not win a point with the serve, you must be sure it is not lost because of a poorly placed serve.

Anticipate Your Opponent's Shot

The beginning player is restricted to playing from a center-court position during a rally because of his or her *inability to anticipate ball movement* and lack of playing skill. Most shots can be hit easily from the center court, and most poorly placed balls rebound to this area. Therefore, it is an ideal location for the novice player.

The experienced player usually is facing an opponent whose shot selection is varied, and ball control allows more skill in court placement.

Rather than playing the *court*, as the beginning player does, the more experienced player plays the *shot*. This means you should anticipate the best return your opponent can hit and begin moving for the ball's predicted path before it is hit.

Anticipating a shot is not always guesswork. Many players signal the kind of shot they are going to make

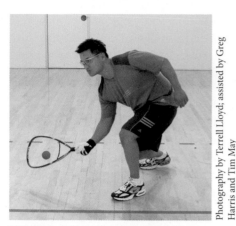

Photography by Terrell Lloyd; assisted by Greg Harris and Tim May

PHOTO 9.2 Racquet Angle Indicating a Return to a Front Corner.

merely by their body position relative to the ball. Because you are watching the ball at all times, you can simultaneously watch your opponent set up to hit the ball. Notice changes in stance (hip and foot placement), and racquet-head angle. Look for any body or racquet position that is consistent with one particular shot (see Photo 9.2). If nothing is apparent but you are beaten continually by one particular return, use the game situation and court position as a guide to when that shot will be used, then move to cover it.

To help anticipate the ball's movement, especially how hard the ball is hit, use your ears as well as your eyes. The sound of the ball hitting the racquet can give you a clue as to the power of the stroke. A strong hit makes a louder sound against the strings of the racquet than does an easy return or a mishit.

Listen to the sound of the hit to anticipate how hard and fast the ball will rebound off the front wall.

In the case where your opponent is caught in the back court and must run quickly to return a soft rebound off the front wall, you should anticipate a hard-hit return. Typically, there is little control over the shot because your opponent is running so quickly to catch up with the ball as it rebounds off the front wall.

It is simply easier to hit the ball with a strong stroke that complements the run.

If your opponent anticipated a soft rebound off the front wall and is waiting for the opportunity to return the ball, either a touch return or hard-hit ball can occur. You will have to make a decision which type of return to cover: either come into the front court or wait for a strong rebound. If you are in this situation, wait as long as possible to return the ball so you can watch where your opponent moves on the court.

Use the Court Wisely

A player's court position can be used to an advantage in two ways: (1) To take away the opponent's best shot—the shot that has a high probability of being a winner, and (2) to keep your opponent moving in the court with the purpose of tiring out the player.

The first use of the court requires that you maintain a court position to either (1) make your opponent's best return shot impossible to hit or (2) place you in the ideal position to hit the ball off this return.

This tactic is important only when your opponent has been successful in scoring consistently off one return. To prevent losing more points to this shot, you must position yourself to make this shot ineffective. An example is to stay to the left of center to discourage a down-the-line shot so you can force a weaker cross-court return.

To be effective, your court position must be fixed before the opponent returns the ball. Otherwise, your court position has not helped you. The purpose of positioning yourself on the court in this manner is to eliminate this shot as one of your opponent's options. If you are successful in discouraging this shot, you must be prepared to move quickly to return a ball hit to another area of the court.

The objective of the second use of the court is to literally keep your opponent running. Shot selection is determined by the other player's weaknesses and also with consideration as to how far your opponent would have to move to get to the ball. For example, if you have just hit the ball to the backhand side, return the ball to the forehand side. Varying placement of the ball short and long is also effective if your opponent has not anticipated the short ball and set up for this return.

Even the most conditioned player will fatigue after long rallies in which the ball must be hit from all parts of the court. This tactic can be especially valuable at the end of the game, when fatigue causes slower reaction and movement times.

Use the Drop Shot

An effective shot for the advanced player that keeps the opponent moving is the drop shot. The drop shot is an offensive shot that requires placement, timing, and deception. Therefore, it is not considered a shot for novice players.

The drop shot can be hit with either a forehand or a backhand stroke. Most players find this shot most successful if it is used from a front-court position. This is true especially when the opponent is caught in the back court.

Often the player is not positioned in the front court for the shot and has to move there from a center-court position with the intent of hitting a drop shot. Therefore, the best ball from which to hit a drop shot is one that rebounds off the back wall and runs to the front court. Consequently, the player must follow the ball into the front court to return it.

The deception in a drop shot is that it looks like any other hard-hit stroke. The opponent expects the ball to rebound quickly off the front wall.

At the point of contact, however, the forward swing is slowed and the face of the racquet is opened. The ball is "kissed" with just enough force to return it to the front. The deadened hit results in a rebound that drops immediately to the floor. If the opponent is in the back court or even the center court, a well-executed drop shot will not be returned.

To ensure success of the drop shot, try to hit the ball to a front corner. If the ball makes contact with both the front wall and a side wall, its movement naturally will be deadened. Thus, a ball hit with too much force will still slow and drop quickly to the floor.

If your opponent follows you to the front court in anticipation of a drop shot, you can still win the point by hitting away at the ball. A hard, low rebound off the front wall will catch your opponent moving in the wrong direction. Using a drop shot or hitting the ball with a strong stroke is determined by your opponent's court position.

Return to the Offensive Position

Because the serve provides the server with the first opportunity to score, the server is considered to be the offensive player. As such, the server initially is in control of the game.

Thus, the receiver's job is to regain the serve and thereby the offense.

The first step in this strategy requires that you move the opponent out of the center-court position. Any of the defensive strokes or a down-the-line or cross-court return will work equally well. The preference for the latter two shots is that they are offensive returns and have the potential for ending the rally immediately.

Neither of these strokes, however, should be hit unless the ball is served at waist level or below.

Balls that are served high off the front wall or that rebound high into the back court (such as the lob or Z-ball) should be hit with your best defensive return.

With any of these returns, the server will be pulled out of the center-court position, which you now can assume. Consequently, you have eliminated the server's offensive court advantage and regained this position yourself.

To make the best return off serves that rebound off the floor high against the back wall, make it a practice to hit the serves as soon as possible after the floor bounce. If you allow the ball to strike the back wall, you must hit the ball as it falls to the floor, possibly close to the corner. Hitting the serve before it touches the back wall usually will give you a better shot opportunity.

Similarly, balls that would run the corner should be taken before the corner is hit. Otherwise, you will face a difficult return. This may mean positioning yourself a step or two closer to the front wall and away from the back wall to catch the bounce.

Obviously, this position will put you at a disadvantage for a short drive serve that rebounds off the side wall directly into your body. But you need to be prepared mentally to return this type of serve before it occurs.

Just like the beginning player, you must plan how you will return the serve rather than just be involved in the play.

Returning to an offensive position can be done in two ways: (1) Hit a winning shot off the return (kill or passing shot), or (2) hit a defensive shot that forces the server to leave the center-court position.

The choice of the return usually depends on the choice of serve. A low ball (below your waist) is a prime candidate for an offensive return; a high ball (above your shoulder) is a prime candidate for a defensive shot. Balls falling in between should either be taken before dropping below shoulder level or be hit after falling below the waist. Balls that rebound off the floor toward the back wall should be taken after the floor bounce, before the wall is hit.

Hit a Winning Shot

A shot can result in a score for one of three reasons: The ball was hit so well that the opponent could not return it even in a proper court position (kill shot), (2) the ball was hit to an area of the court that the opponent could not reach in time to return the ball (passing shot), or (3) the opponent just missed the ball—an unforced error.

The third reason for a score may be related to your play only if you have consistently hit for long rallies with a mix of offensive and defensive shots to tire the opposing player.

Otherwise, unforced errors must be considered a result of a mental lapse on your opponent's part, and you cannot take credit for the point.

The first and second reasons for a winning shot depend upon your play. To hit a winning shot, you must be aggressive. Always move quickly to the ball, and align yourself correctly for the proper hit. Do not wait for the ball to come to you or be satisfied with hitting the ball when it happens to be within reach if you can maneuver for a better shot.

There are three times when you can consider hitting the ball as it rebounds from the front wall (see Chapter 4). Which you choose depends on how aggressively you are playing and whether you want to speed up or slow down the game.

The first is after the ball rebounds off the front wall and before it touches the floor. This is called a **volley**.

Any shot can be hit as a volley with either a forehand or a backhand stroke. Ideally, you must still pivot when volleying the ball, to ensure a proper stroke on the return.

A volleyed ball, however, is often a mishit because the player has not set up properly for a defensive or offensive shot. Thus, the ball is hit with an unorthodox stroke and loses its effectiveness. This happens because of the ball's quick rebound off the front wall, which allows little time to set up properly for the return.

Therefore, hitting a good volley is not as dependent upon moving to the ball as it is upon the ball rebounding to the appropriate court position to allow you time to hit it. Consequently, every ball is not a good prospect for a volley return.

Unfortunately, beginning players often volley a return to avoid (1) moving to a correct position to hit a ball, or (2) returning balls that would rebound off the back wall. Experienced players volley a return with one of three strategies in mind: (1) to change the pace of the game by speeding up the return to the front wall, (2) to avoid having the ball rebound into a court position (corner) that would make a strong return impossible, or (3) to force an opponent to hit a return before he or she can set up properly for the ball.

The third strategy is executed most effectively if the ball is returned directly to the opponent. As a result of this return, the opponent typically is handcuffed. The ball rebounds so quickly to the player's position that there is no time to get the racquet head moving to hit the ball. Therefore, the experienced player chooses to hit a volley for a strategic reason rather than because the ball merely rebounds within reach.

Beginning players hitting a volley with an overhead stroke should direct the ball either to the ceiling for a defensive shot or directly to the front wall in an attempt to pass the opponent. More experienced players may return an overhead kill.

A volleyed ball hit from a position low off the floor provides an opportunity to hit a kill shot return.

Even beginning players may attempt this offensive volley with a low rebounding ball, especially if they are holding a center- or midcourt position.

If you choose to let the ball bounce, it may be hit immediately after touching the floor as it passes between your shoelaces and knee, or finally after the height of the arc is reached and the ball is falling to the floor, passing again through this same area. Aggressive players try to take most balls on the skip or short hop, just after the floor is hit. This also works to speed up play and may catch the opponent out of court position. In addition, it offers the advantage of being at the right position from which to hit a kill shot.

Waiting until the ball arcs and is falling for the second time to the floor gives you more time to set up for the shot, and your opponent more time to set up for the return. Therefore, hitting the ball at this point should be done primarily by the beginning player who reacts slowly to the ball, or by the experienced player who is trying to slow down the game.

Regardless of where you are when you hit the ball or what kind of ball you hit, move to cut off your opponent's anticipated return after you hit the ball. There, you will be the least vulnerable to your opponent's next shot, and you can begin to set up for another winning return.

A Good Defense May Be the Best Offense

Every player will meet someone who is a match against the best serves or who can anticipate the ball's movement in the court and can score at will. Often this is the case when a beginning player plays a more experienced player. As a result, because of the speed and power of his or her strokes, the more experienced player seems to be playing in a different time zone.

The only way to make a game of this situation is to try to outmaneuver the power. This can be done in three ways: (1) slow the ball and the tempo of the game by waiting to hit the ball just before the second bounce, (2) use defensive return shots to the opponent's weak side and hit garbage serves, and (3) keep your opponent out of the center court by hitting balls wide of the midline.

Trying to outgun power usually leads to a sloppy game, referred to as Battleball (see Chapter 7). Using a strategy that does not give your opponent anything good to hit or a court position from which to hit it may eliminate power as a factor. Thus, the best offense for even some experienced players against a power player is a good defensive game. It may not have the spark and strong rallies of a power game, but the weaker player who is the tactician will have a chance to score.

This is not to imply that the player can never hit offensive shots, but rather, that these shots should be attempted only when there is a high probability of success. Indeed, the defensive game should be used to tire the opponent by moving him or her around the court, frustrating him or her into an unforced error, or soliciting a weak return that sets up your offensive shot.

The name of this game is patience—patience to endure the long rallies and wait for your opening to an offensive position. Above all, to use this strategy effectively, you must be careful never to hit a low ball to your opponent's strong side, because that is just the opportunity needed to begin a power game.

Play the Weakness

Every player has a weakness—a shot the player would prefer not to hit. Your job is to find that weakness and take advantage of it if you can.

If the opponent does not appear to have a weakness, create one through ball placement and court position. A player who is running to hit a ball constantly will fatigue no matter how well conditioned, so keep the ball moving. If the player is much

stronger than you, go for broke. Try to hit everything and anything, even the best kill shot. If you concede the shot, the point is lost; if you try for the ball, you may return just a few and stop a rally. If nothing else, Mr. or Ms. Sharpshooter may think twice about the choice of hits, knowing that you came close to returning a ball. This hesitancy may cause some mishits and provide better opportunities for making offensive returns.

To have any hope that this strategy will succeed, give yourself the best chance for hitting a winner. Never hit the ball and hold court position. *Move* to cut off the return, and *hustle*. If this strategy doesn't work, at least you put up a fight!

Know Your Own Capabilities

Knowing your opponent's weaknesses is only half of what you need to know to win at racquetball. You also need to know your own capabilities and strengths. Even the best players must play to their strengths and try to play around their weaknesses.

Hitting shots that are strategically smart but low-percentage returns for you will only give away points. Knowing what should be done and the ability to execute it are two different skills. At higher levels of the game, points should be won because of skill, not lost because of lack of skill.

The best way to learn your capabilities is during practice. If you cannot consistently hit a shot during practice, you will be unlikely to execute the shot well during a game. Games are not the time to develop skills, but to exhibit them. It is during practice that you can determine what your capabilities are and what weaknesses you need to work on.

As a result, practice must be structured beginning with the basics and working to more advanced skills. The tendency is to begin to practice with forehand strokes. Typically, however, backhand strokes are weaker. Whichever is true, it is a better use of your time to begin working on the weakest part of your game first when you are fresh and concentrating fully.

If you consistently mishit a ball, ask a local pro or an advanced racquetball player to watch you play.

Repeating an incorrect stroke or court position will reinforce ineffective play. Correct errors early in your playing career, or you will be struggling to get rid of these bad habits as you are trying to improve your skills. Once you know what your capabilities are, you can easily prepare to use your best shots during play. Developing a game plan around these strengths will make the game more enjoyable and also allow you to play your best.

POINTS *to* REMEMBER

Play an offensive game, plan your shots, and move your opponent around the court to set up your best return.

Vary your serves by changing the force of the hit, the angle off the front wall, and where the ball rebounds behind the short line.

Anticipate your opponent's shot, and move to a court position to block it or set up for the return.

Use defensive shots from the back-court position and offensive returns from a center- or front-court position.

Keep your opponent away from a center-court position by hitting the ball wide of the midline of the court and into the back corners.

When you are tired, hit harder and move faster.

When playing a stronger opponent, play a defensive game and slow the tempo of play.

Control the Rally

The thinking strategy requires that you seek to control each rally regardless of whether you served or received the serve. Obviously, if you are the server, you should set the tone for the rally by serving your best. If you are receiving the serve, as previously stated, your first objective should be to minimally move into an offensive court position as a result of your return of serve.

Once you have achieved a center-court position, you have the potential to control the rally, but you can accomplish this only if you take advantage of your court position. Your goal from this position is to hit a winning shot. Unlike the non-thinking strategy—in which most points are scored because of an opponent's error—you should earn the point because of your play.

If your opponent is also hitting from the center court, balls hit hard to the front wall give him or her little time to react. This is especially true if a passing shot is hit. A down-the-line pass or a cross-court pass can be equally effective.

Be aware, however, that this strategy also can be used on you! Be aggressive and make this play first. A well-placed, front wall–straight-in kill shot toward the side wall farthest from your opponent is almost always effective if executed correctly.

If your opponent is caught in the front court, a hard-hit ball placed to rebound directly back into his or her body, as described with a volley, often handcuffs your opponent into a mishit. A kill shot, however, may not be effective in this situation because your opponent will be in a good position to return your shot with another kill.

Your other choice would be a passing shot that dies in the back court before a return is made. Be careful not to hit this ball so hard that it rebounds off the back wall into a center-court position. If this is a common mistake of yours, hit the passing shot low to the front wall. This way, even if it rebounds off the back wall, it will be difficult to return from the back court. Also, you may mishit the ball and actually hit a kill shot!

Another key to controlling the rally when your opponent is in the center or front court is to keep the ball moving fast and away from where he or she is standing. Don't prolong the rally with slow-moving balls. Your goal is to win a point or the serve as quickly as possible. The only time you should hit a defensive shot from this position is when your opponent is stronger, faster, and has more skill. Then, hitting a defensive return that forces him or her to move into a back-court position may allow you to be the only player positioned to end the rally with an offensive shot.

If your opponent is in the back court, your options are numerous. You can return a softly hit ball to the front wall or make a hard-hit kill. You can hit defensive shots to force your opponent to remain in that position. The only shot not available to use is a passing shot.

If you are the player forced into a back-court position and your opponent is in front of you, you should use a defensive shot or passing shot. Of course, if your kill shot is effective from this position and you have confidence in its success, you might as well try to end the rally.

Otherwise, work to move your opponent out of an offensive court position so you may take the center court and, with it, control of the rally.

If both of you are in the back court and your opponent hits a good defensive shot, don't try to end the rally by forcing an offensive return. Rather, respond to a well-placed defensive shot with another well-placed defensive shot. Patience is key at this point. Wait until you have a better offensive opportunity or can create one. This opportunity depends upon what shot is given to you as well as where your opponent is on the court.

If you find yourself in the front court and your opponent is behind you, a pinch kill usually ends the rally if it is hit correctly. If you are caught too close to the front wall, you may want to use a defensive shot to force your opponent back and give you time to reposition yourself into a better court position. This is a difficult shot and requires quick movement on your part. Most importantly, do not turn to face the back wall and run into position, as you would be exposing yourself to a direct frontal hit from your opponent's return. Run backward to the desired court position. Getting hit in the back is not nearly as destructive as getting hit in the face.

If you can contol your opponent's court position, you can control the rally and, with it, the outcome of the game. This requires a thinking strategy.

CHECKPOINTS

Answers are located on page 141.

1. To maintain an offensive center-court position, you can:
   a. return the ball wide of center.
   b. hit a high rebound into the back court.
   c. hit a down-the-line shot.
   d. all of the above.

2. You have the best chance of winning if you:
   a. hustle.
   b. anticipate your opponent's shot.
   c. play to your opponent's weakness.
   d. all of the above.

3. The thinking strategy:
   a. relies on strategies to win points, including offensive shots.
   b. should be used before the non-thinking strategy, which is typically more spontaneous.
   c. allows the opponent to stay in the center court.
   d. plays to the opponent's strengths but wins as a result of outthinking him or her.

4. The "right" serve is defined as:
   a. a legal serve.
   b. one in which an offensive shot is not returned.
   c. one to the opponent's back hand.
   d. one that is hit down the middle of the court.

5. With the serve, you:
   a. can control the game.
   b have the most opportunities to lose points.
   c. are at the mercy of your opponent's strength and skill.
   d. should have a goal of simply putting the ball in play.

6. Variety can be added to the serve by:
   a. hitting the ball softly so it hits the floor in front of the service box.
   b. having the ball rebound off the ceiling after hitting the front wall.
   c. both a and b.
   d. neither a nor b.

7. The same basic serve can be hit:
   a. to the forehand or backhand side.
   b. short or long.
   c. high or low.
   d. hard or soft.
   e. all of the above.

8. A low, hard hit serve is:
   a. more difficult to control.
   b. more effective in forcing a poor return.
   c. effective if the strengths of your game out number the strengths of your opponent.
   d. two of the above.
   e. all of the above.

9. A primary difference between a beginning racquetball player and an experienced one is:
   a. the experienced player relies on defensive shots to win the point.
   b. the experienced player anticipates the ball's movement and plays the ball rather than the court.
   c. the beginning player listens for the sound of the ball hitting the racquet, while the experienced player turns and watches the play.
   d. two of the above.
   e. all of the above.

10. If your opponent appears fatigued:
    a. hit the serve slower so he or she will have their timing off to return the ball.
    b. keep returning the ball to the same area of the court to try tire his or her arm.
    c. try to finish the rally as quickly as possible.
    d. it is a good time to hit a drop shot if your opponent is in the back-court areas.

11. When receiving a serve:
    a. you are on the defensive and need to work to regain the serve and an offensive position.
    b. try to minimally return the serve so that your opponent must leave the center court position.
    c. you can make a defensive or offensive shot.
    d. two of the above.
    e. all of the above.

12. To play aggressively means you:
    a. take your time and wait for the ball.
    b. hit a volley to force your opponent's return before he or she is prepared to do so.
    c. keep the ball in play until your opponent makes an error.
    d. always wait and hit the ball at the last possible moment to take your opponent by surprise.

13. Which of the following is true:
    a. every player has a weakness.
    b. playing a more skilled player may require a patient, defensive game.
    c. when playing a more skilled player, never hit an offensive shot because they will always return it.
    d. two of the above.
    e. all of the above.

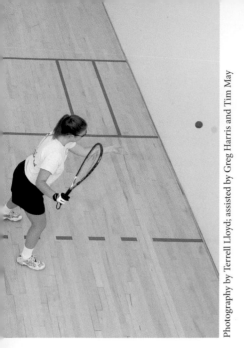

Photography by Terrell Lloyd; assisted by Greg Harris and Tim May

10

Drills for the Player

Racquetball drills help the beginning player develop the skills necessary to play the game, and they give the experienced player opportunities to practice and sharpen all shots. Drills also may be part of your warm-up routine to help you get the feel for the court and the ball's movement, as well as to help your body adjust to exercise.

The following drills were designed to provide opportunities for players to work on the strokes and shots used most often in game situations. Evaluative measures accompany some drills to help you determine your proficiency with that skill and when you will be ready to incorporate it into your game plan. The drills presented can be used to practice the most basic skills to playing modified games with an opponent. The beginning player can either start with the first drill and work through to the simulated games or pick the drills that use the skills that are most difficult.

In all drills, starting the ball in play properly is critical. The ball can be either dropped to the floor or tossed against a wall. You must drop the ball in front of your forward foot so you can step into the stroke when contacting the ball. If the ball

is tossed to a wall, position yourself so the rebound falls in front of your body position. This will allow you to step forward to meet the ball. The wrong ball toss will result in learning to hit a ball that is positioned improperly in relation to your body.

Scoring Scales

Scoring scales are presented in selected drills. The illustrations accompanying these drills indicate the size of the target area (one or two feet) and the points allotted to each target zone (five, three, or one). Balls in the targeted area can be scored by making a best guess or by placing small pieces of masking tape on the floor and walls to outline the areas. Balls that hit a line between two point areas should be given the lower of the two scores. A legal shot not hitting the target area is scored zero points.

Although the target points are somewhat arbitrary, they do identify, through points scored, the accuracy and placement of your shots. In general, the percentages listed on Table 10.1 can be used to determine the effectiveness of your returns and serves.

TABLE 10.1
Scoring Scales

Category	Percent	Use
Excellent	90 – 100	"Bread and butter" shot; use this shot whenever your strategy dictates
Good	75 – 89	Consistent enough to use to vary your shots; a dependable shot in a game in which you are in control
Average	50 – 74	Be careful—you may miss this shot half of the time; not the shot to choose when the game is close, but a good shot to practice when you can afford to lose some points
Below Average	below 50	POISON!—Do not hit this in a game situation because you will miss it more than half of the time

DRILL 1

Watching the Game

Purpose: To develop a concept of how racquetball is played and the use of offensive and defensive shots during the game.

Method: Go to a court with an observation area and watch experienced players play racquetball. Count the number of offensive and defensive shots each player uses.

DRILL 2

Forehand Shots

Purpose: To practice hitting a forehand shot to the back corners of the court from three primary areas of the floor.

Method: Hit eight balls each from the mid-, center-, and back-court positions (see Figure 10.1). From each position, hit four balls to the back right corner and four balls to the back left corner. Hit the ball after you've dropped it to the floor.

DRILL 3

Backhand Shots

Purpose: To practice hitting a backhand shot to the back corners of the court from three primary areas of the floor.

Method: Hit eight balls each from the mid-, center-, and back-court positions

(see Figure 10.1). From each position, hit four balls to the back right corner and four balls to the back left corner. Hit the ball after you've dropped it to the floor.

DRILL 4

Forehand and Backhand Shots from Side-Wall Toss

Purpose: To practice hitting forehand and backhand shots to the back corners of the court from a ball bouncing off the side wall.

Method: Stand with your hips pivoted and facing the side wall appropriate for either a forehand or a backhand stroke. Using an underhand toss, toss the ball into the side wall (see Photo 10.1).

After the rebound and the first bounce off the floor, hit the ball to a back corner of the court. Hit eight balls from each of the three court positions, four to each corner, then repeat eight shots each from the same court positions with the other stroke.

DRILL 5

Suicide Drill

Purpose: To develop muscular endurance and anaerobic capacity, and to practice moving to the ball and returning it to the front wall.

Method: Begin in the center court, and after dropping the ball, hit it to the front wall. Continue to return the ball

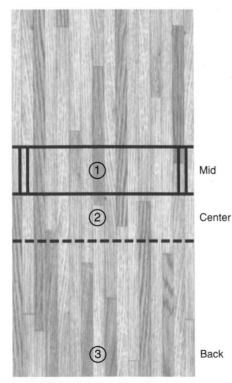

FIGURE 10.1 Hitting Positions for Stroking Drill.

Mid ①

Center ②

Back ③

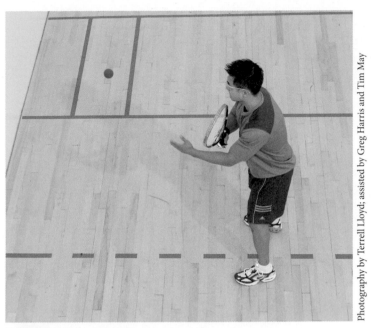

PHOTO 10.1 Underhand Toss Off the Side Wall.

Photography by Terrell Lloyd; assisted by Greg Harris and Tim May

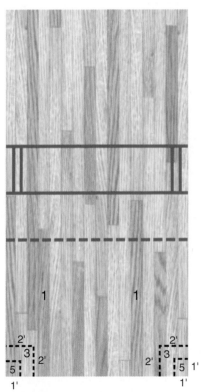

FIGURE 10.2 Scoring Area for the Lob and High-Z Serving Drill.

as quickly as you can, hitting all balls regardless of their court position or the number of times the ball has bounced off the floor. Work at positioning yourself correctly for each hit. Continue this drill for 2-minute intervals, allowing yourself to rest 30 seconds to a minute after each hitting session. Repeat the drill 10 times. Record the number of balls hit during each two-minute interval.

DRILL 6

30-Second Drill

Purpose: To teach the player to react quickly to the ball's court position and improve his or her movement time, and to work on ball control.

Method: Begin in a center-court position. Drop the ball and return it

to the front wall. Continue to return the ball off the rebound, counting the number of times the ball is returned in 30 seconds. Count only the shots that would be legal returns in a game. Do this drill at least every other practice session. Try to improve one to three shots each time.

DRILL 7

Serving Drill—Lob and High-Z

Purpose: To practice hitting lob and high-Z serves correctly and accurately to a back-corner court position.

Method: Standing close to the center of the service zone, hit 10 lob serves to the right back corner of the court to the designated target area. Score each serve as indicated in Figure 10.2.

Give one point to a legal serve if it lands on the correct side of the court and not in the back corner.

Total the points. Refer to the scoring scale to determine the accuracy of this serve. Total points possible: 50 points.

Repeat this drill with the lob serve to the left back corner and the target area. Score and evaluate. Total points: 50.

(Note: For a lob hit with a backhand stroke, you may move in the service area toward the backhand side wall.)

Repeat both parts of this drill using a high-Z serve. Total points possible for each part: 50 points.

Scoring Scale

	Points
Excellent	45–50
Good	39–44
Average	25–38
Below Average	fewer than 25

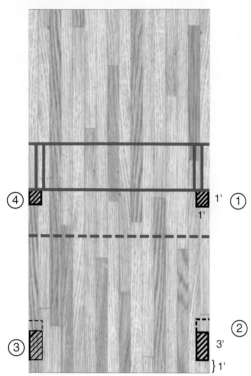

FIGURE 10.3   Scoring Area for the Drive Serve.

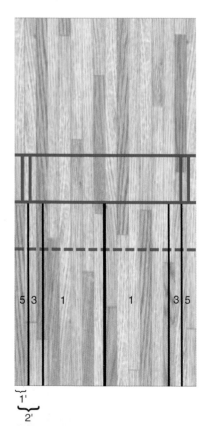

FIGURE 10.4   Scoring Area for the Back-wall Drill.

DRILL 8

Serving Drills—Drive Serve

Purpose: To develop accuracy in your drive serve and be able to drive serve to a variety of court positions.

Method: From the center of the service zone, hit three drive serves to each of the four designated court positions (see Figure 10.3). Repeat the circuit three times. Score one point for each correct placement. Total points possible: 36. (Note: You can total points scored to each designated area to indicate your most accurate placement. Total points to each area: 9.)

Scoring Scale

	Points
Excellent	32–36
Good	27–31
Average	18–26
Below Average	fewer than 18

DRILL 9

Defensive Shots— Lob, Ceiling, High-Z, Around-the-Wall

Purpose: To practice hitting a defensive shot from two court positions and develop accuracy placing the ball.

Method: Using a dropped ball, hit each defensive shot 10 times, from center- and back-court positions (5 to each corner).

Use the same target area as designated for the lob and high-Z serves. Total points possible for each serve from each position: 50. To vary this drill, begin the defensive shot with a side-wall toss.

Scoring Scale

	Points
Excellent	45–50
Good	39–44
Average	25–38
Below Average	fewer than 25

DRILL 10

Back-Wall Drill

Purpose: To practice hitting balls rebounding off the back wall and accurately returning them wide of the midline in a back-court area.

Method: Standing in the back court, toss balls into the back wall to rebound for a forehand stroke. Hit 10 balls, returning each to the front. Score the rebound in the designated area (see Figure 10.4). Total points possible: 50.

Repeat the drill using a ball toss to your backhand side, and return the balls with a backhand stroke. Total points possible: 50.

Scoring Scale

	Points
Excellent	45–50
Good	39–44
Average	25–38
Below Average	fewer than 25

DRILL 11

Corner Return

Purpose: To practice hitting balls after they have rebounded from a back corner and accurately returning them into a back-court position wide of the midline.

Method: Standing in the back court, toss a ball to your forehand side to rebound either from the back wall to a side wall or in the opposite direction (see Figures 10.5 and 10.6). Return 10 balls with your forehand stroke, then turn and toss 10 balls to the opposite side or back wall for a backhand return (see Figure 10.6). Hit each ball to rebound into a back-court position and wide of the midline of the court. Score each return with the same designated target area used for the back-wall returns.

Total points possible for each stroke: 50.

Scoring Scale

	Points
Excellent	45–50
Good	39–44
Average	25–38
Below Average	fewer than 25

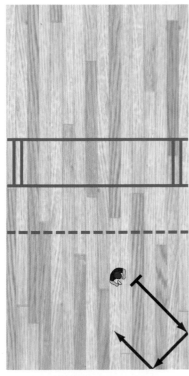

Tossed Ball

FIGURE 10.5   Path of a Tossed Ball for the Corner Hit Drill—Side Wall Toss.

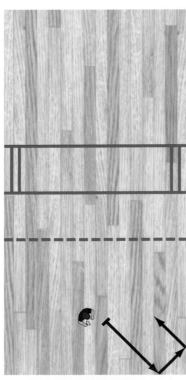

Tossed Ball

FIGURE 10.6   Path of a Tossed Ball for the Corner Hit Drill—Back Wall Toss.

Repeat Ceiling Shots

Purpose: To practice hitting balls rebounding off the back wall and accurately returning them with a defensive shot wide of the midline in a backcourt area.

Method: Standing in the back court, toss balls into the back wall to rebound for a forehand stroke. Hit 10 balls, returning each with a ceiling-front wall shot. Score the rebound in the designated area.

Total points possible: 50.

Repeat the drill using a ball toss to your backhand side, and return the balls with a backhand stroke. Total points possible: 50.

Scoring Scale

	Points
Excellent	45–50
Good	39–44
Average	25–38
Below Average	fewer than 25

DRILL 13

Offensive Shots— Passing

Purpose: To practice hitting passing shots from two court positions and accurately directing them to one of two court areas.

Method: Using a side-wall toss to your forehand side, hit 10 passing shots from the court position identified in Figures 10.7 and 10.8. Return the ball into the shaded area of the figure. Score one point for each successful return. Total points possible: 10.

Repeat the drill using a backhand stroke.

Total points possible: 10.

Scoring Scale

	Points
Excellent	9–10
Good	7–8
Average	5–6
Below Average	fewer than 5

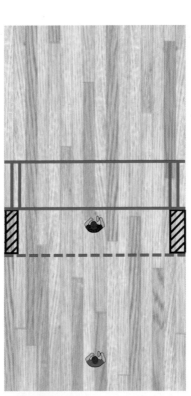

FIGURE 10.7   Target Area for a Passing Shot from a Back-court Position.

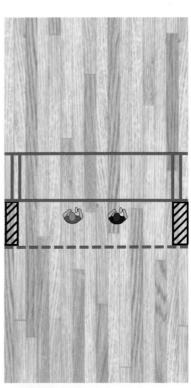

FIGURE 10.8   Target Area for a Passing Shot from a Center-court Position.

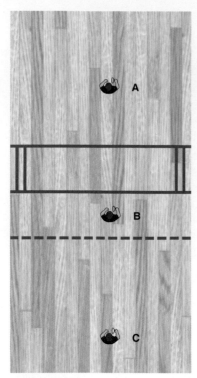

FIGURE 10.9 Hitting Positions for the Kill Shot Drill.

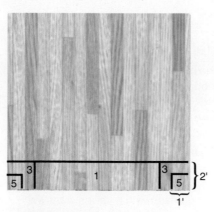

FIGURE 10.10 Scoring Area for the Kill Shot Drill.

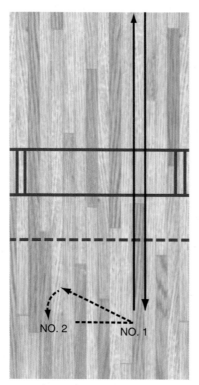

FIGURE 10.11 Rally Drill to Avoid Collisions on the Court.

Offensive Shots—Kill

Purpose: To practice hitting accurate kill shots from three court positions.

Method: Dropping the ball to your forehand side, hit 10 kill shots from each court position: A, B, and C (see Figure 10.9). Score each position separately using a front-wall target area (see Figure 10.10). Use corner and pinch kill shots. Total points possible: 50.

Repeat the drill using a drop to your backhand side. Total points possible: 50 from each court position. This drill can be varied by using a side-wall toss to put the ball in play.

Scoring Scale

	Points
Excellent	45–50
Good	39–44
Average	25–38
Below Average	fewer than 25

Rally Drill—Hit and Move

Purpose: To practice hitting a ball and moving away from the rebound to avoid colliding with your opponent on the court.

Method: Standing side by side with your opponent in the back court, the player on the right side of the court hits a ball straight into the front wall. After hitting, this player moves to the left and out of the way of the opponent moving toward the ball (see Figure 10.11). The ball is again returned straight into the front wall, and the positions are again reversed.

Continue this rotation until the ball is missed.

Mini-game

Purpose: To give players a chance to practice serving and returning the serve.

Method: Each player serves five times and then rotates to the back court to be the receiver. The game is to 15 points, and a point is scored by either player on each serve regardless of whether he or she was serving.

Defensive Return Game

Purpose: To practice hitting a defensive shot off any serve.

Method: Only the server scores. The server must use a drive serve, and the receiver a ceiling or other defensive return. If the receiver does not use this type of return, the server scores a point. If the drive serve is not hit, a side-out occurs. Variation: Change the type of serve required to be hit, or specify exactly which defensive shot is to be returned.

Game Warm-up Drill

Purpose: To provide a method for warming up before a game.

Method: Begin by standing side by side with your opponent just behind the short line (see Photo 10.2). Practice hitting forehand strokes to the front wall. After several minutes, move two-thirds of the way to the back wall and practice ceiling shots from this position. Finally, back up to the back wall and hit offensive and defensive returns to the front wall from a ball toss off the back wall.

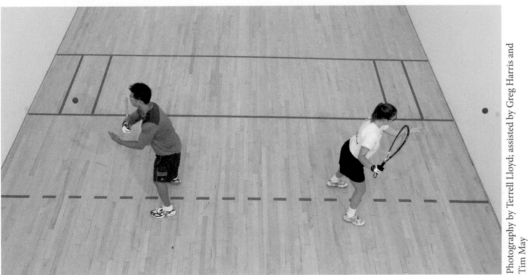

Photography by Terrell Lloyd; assisted by Greg Harris and Tim May

PHOTO 10.2   Players Warming Up Before a Game.

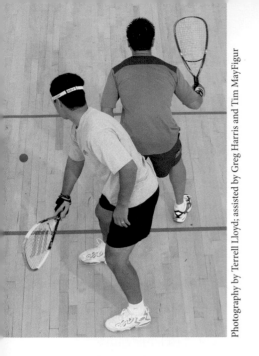

Photography by Terrell Lloyd; assisted by Greg Harris and Tim MayFigur

Court Etiquette, Interpreting Rules, and Strategy

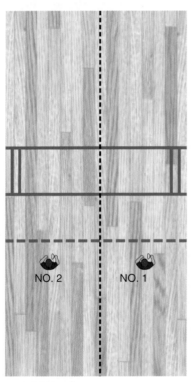

FIGURE 11.1 Court Divided in Length for Warm-up.

As in all sports activities, courtesy is involved in competitive racquetball. We need to understand and interpret the rules of the game in a fair and objective manner. With two individuals enclosed in a space of 20 feet by 40 feet by 20 feet, there is little room for disagreement.

The possibility of injury and negative feelings increases if every courtesy is not extended to the opponent and if the rules are not complied with meticulously.

Prior to the Start

Prior to the start of the match, the court must be shared by players executing the shots to be used in the match. In that warm-up, each player should control ball placement to avoid interfering with the opponent. The court should be divided in length, and all shots should be hit within that boundary (see Figure 11.1 and Photo 11.1).

During the warm-up, players should hit only shots they can control, and they should be considerate if the opponent retrieves a ball from the front of the court. Stopping execution of a shot if the opponent walks in front of you and returning a ball to an opponent by bouncing the ball to the player are expectations related to both etiquette and safety (see Photos 11.2 and 11.3).

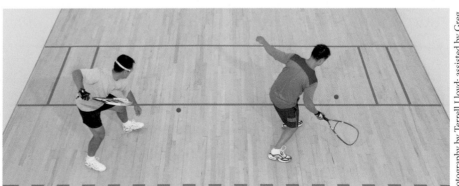

PHOTO 11.1 Two Players Warming Up Side by Side.

Photography by Terrell Lloyd; assisted by Greg Harris and Tim May

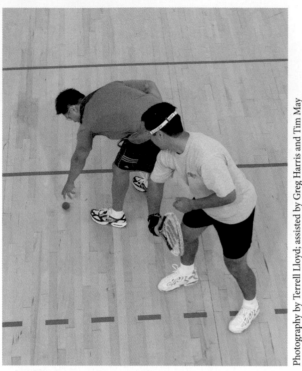

Photography by Terrell Lloyd; assisted by Greg Harris and Tim May

PHOTO 11.2   Stopping Execution of Warm-up Shot When a Player Walks in Front of Another Player.

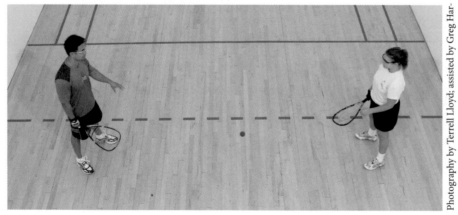

Photography by Terrell Lloyd; assisted by Greg Harris and Tim May

PHOTO 11.3   Bouncing the Ball Back to Opponent When Warming Up.

About the Rally, Game and Match, Serving, and Ball in Play

Instituting proper etiquette and interpretation of the rules during the game is crucial to acceptable play.

Some of the rules are quite simple, yet the beginning player sometimes does not respond initially to the obvious and has to be informed of a rule that most experienced players take for granted.

Rally, Points, and Outs

A rally occurs once the ball is placed in play by a serve, and it continues until a player fails to hit the front wall prior to the ball striking the floor, when the ball touches the floor twice, or as a result of a hinder. Points are scored (see Appendix, Rule 1.4, Points and Outs) only by the serving side at the conclusion of a rally.

A serve lost following a rally is called a **sideout** in singles, and a **handout** in doubles. The objective of racquetball is to win each rally by serving or returning serve until the opponent fails to keep the ball in play (see Appendix, Rule 1.3, Objective).

Game and Match

Keeping score is one of those rules that is taken for granted, yet it should be explained. A game is won when the first player reaches 15 points; thus, a score of 15–14 is a legal game. To win a match in most situations requires you to win the best of three games. If each player has won one game, the third game is played to 11 points, again with the need to win by only one point (see Appendix, Rule 1.5, Match, Game, Tiebreaker). In class situations, students may discover that games are played to an assortment of final points to accommodate class procedure.

Serving

Specific *rules govern the service* in racquetball (see Appendix, Rule 3.1, Serve). Determining who serves first

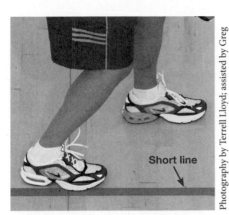

PHOTO 11.4 Legal Position of Server in Relation to Serving Zone.

is done with a coin toss or, in casual play, "lagging" (select a target and the closest to hitting the target serves first) for serve.

The winner of the coin toss elects to receive or serve in the first game, and the second game begins in reverse order. If a tiebreaker is required, the player with the most total points will have the option of serving or receiving (a tie requires another coin flip or "lag").

To begin play, the server must stand between the short line and the service line—an area commonly called the service zone, defined as the back of the paint of the short line and the front of the service line paint (go back to Figure 1.1 in Chapter 1 to check out the service zone). No part of either foot may fully extend beyond either line of the service zone; however, stepping *on* the line is allowed (see Photo 11.4).

To initiate a serve, the player must drop the ball and then strike it with the racquet after the ball rebounds off the floor. Following racquet contact on the serve, the ball must strike the front wall first on the fly and then carry beyond the short line. The ball must strike the floor beyond the short line before hitting the back wall, ceiling, or more than one side wall.

A screen serve, an illegal drive serve, and a serve that strikes the front wall on the fly and doesn't carry beyond the short line are all fault serves. Serves that hit two or more side walls, the back wall on the fly, and the ceiling on the fly are also fault serves. Altogether there are 10 fault serves (see Appendix, Rule 3.9, Fault Serves). Common terms for a fault include a "short" for a serve that doesn't carry past the short line, a "long" for a ball that hits the back wall on the fly, and "three-wall" for a serve that hits more than one side wall on the fly (see Figures 11.2, 11.3, and 11.4).

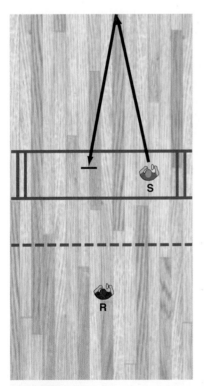

FIGURE 11.2 Short-serve Fault.

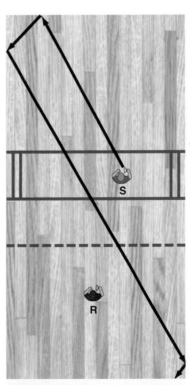

FIGURE 11.3 Three-wall Fault.

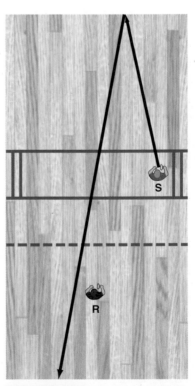

FIGURE 11.4 Long-serve Fault.

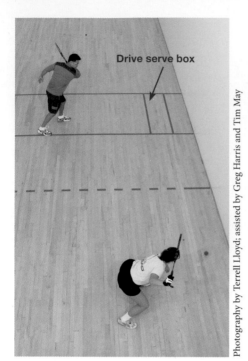

PHOTO 11.5   Drive-serve Box.

Photography by Terrell Lloyd; assisted by Greg Harris and Tim May

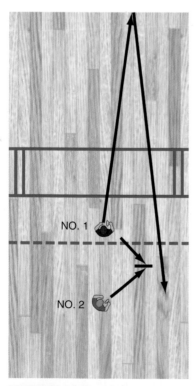

FIGURE 11.5   Blocking an Opponent in Back Court: A Penalty Hinder.

The fault serve as an illegal drive serve deserves special mention. There is a **drive serve zone** (see Appendix, Rule 3.6, Drive Service Zones) consisting of two drive serve lines, each three feet from the side wall, located in the service zone.

The server may drive serve to the same side of the court from where the serve is initiated as long as the start and finish of the server's serve motion take place outside of the three-foot drive serve box (see Photo 11.5). A second serve opportunity is provided following all fault serves.

An **out serve** signifies the loss of serve, which occurs when the ball does not hit the front wall on the fly after the server hits the ball, or when two faults are served in succession.

Additional out serves include an out-of-court serve, a missed serve attempt, a crotch serve off the front wall, a touched serve, a fake balk serve, an illegal hit, a safety zone violation with the server or doubles partner entering the zone before the serve crosses the short line, and a serve striking a partner who is standing outside the doubles box in a doubles match (see Appendix, Rule 3.10, Out Serves).

Calling the score prior to every serve is expected in a racquetball match. The server calls the score.

The receiver, at this point, may express disagreement with the score or prepare to receive the next serve.

Ball in Play

Once the ball is in play, each of the players (in singles) must hit it alternately.

The ultimate goal of either player is to hit the ball so it strikes the front wall before hitting the floor. A ball can hit the back wall, followed by the ceiling and side walls, as long as it eventually gets to the front wall before touching the floor.

A server continues the serve for each point played until two faults are hit in succession, an out serve is made, or the server cannot return the opponent's shot in a legal manner (not returning the ball to the front wall before it strikes the floor, hitting after the second bounce, or committing a point hinder). A return-of-serve player remains in that situation until the serving opponent has made one of the abovementioned errors.

Hinders

When interpreting the rules, hinders have to be discussed in detail. The two basic types of hinders in racquetball are: (1) penalty hinders, usually intentional acts to prevent an opponent from a fair try at hitting the ball, and (2) replay hinders (commonly-called hinders), which are accidental, associated with preventing the opponent from having a fair chance at the ball.

Penalty hinders are usually called on a player who intentionally moves in the path of an opponent to prevent the opponent from hitting the ball or seeing it clearly. Penalty hinders penalize the offending player by a loss of the rally.

Experienced players are quite skilled at committing a penalty hinder called **blocking**. The player committing the infraction may hit a shot from an "up" position and then set up to block the movement of the opponent in a "back" position (see Figure 11.5). The movement is subtle and discourages the opponent from attempting to reach the ball, as the opponent is in a "back" position.

There are countless penalty hinders in racquetball (see Appendix, Rule 3.15, Penalty Hinders).

The player who simply will not move to permit an opponent

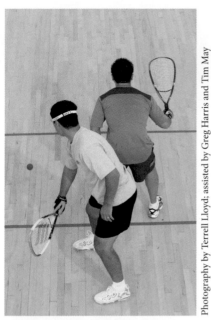

PHOTO 11.6   A player Who Doesn't Move Out of the Way: A Penalty Hinder.

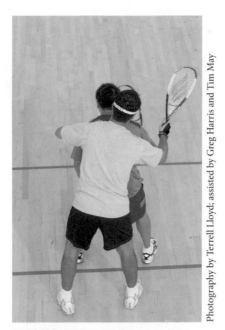

PHOTO 11.7   A Player Moving Too Close to a Player Attempting a Shot: A Penalty Hinder.

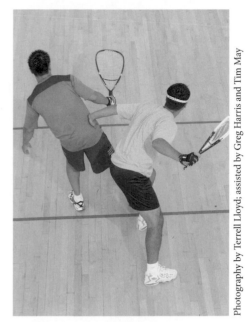

PHOTO 11.8   A Player Pushing an Opponent to Get a Ball: A Penalty Hinder.

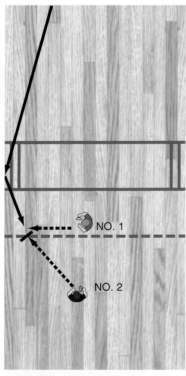

FIGURE 11.6   Moving Into Opponent's Path: A Penalty Hinder.

access to the ball is one example (see Photo 11.6). A second example is a player who will move next to an opponent attempting a full-swing shot. That opponent will not be able to complete the swing because of the position of the other player (see Photo 11.7). A third example is a player pushing or shoving an opponent as a means of gaining impetus to move to reach a ball. Pushing off an opponent gives an unfair advantage, as it may place the opponent in an off-balance position for the next shot (see Photo 11.8).

A fourth distinct violation associated with penalty hinders is intentionally moving the body into the path of the return shot of an opponent. If an opponent strikes the ball from a "back" position and the "up" player (recognizing that the shot would put that player at a great disadvantage for a return) moves into the path of the ball, the call is a penalty hinder (see Figure 11.6).

Replay hinders occur as part of the action of the game and happen without planned effort (see

Appendix, Rule 3.14, Replay Hinders). One example of this is when the ball strikes an irregular portion of the court, such as an edge of the door (see Photo 11.9), a can placed in the corner of the court (see Photo 11.10), or any other part of the court that would impede the progress of play.

Other examples of replay hinders are (1) a player being hit by an opponent's shot prior to the ball striking the front wall (see Figure 11.7); (2) a ball that is "screened" so the opponent cannot see the ball clearly (see Photo 11.11); and (3) a ball that goes between the opponent's legs (see Photo 11.12), distracting the player hitting the ball (not always a hinder, depending on player positioning and proximity of players).

In addition, when two players collide while attempting to move out of the way of each other or the ball (see Photo 11.13) or attempting to reach the ball, play is stopped and a hinder is called. A final hinder is called any time a player about to execute a

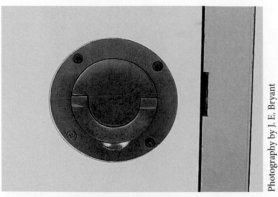

Photography by J. E. Bryant

PHOTO 11.9   Ball Hitting Edge of Door: A
Replay Hinder.

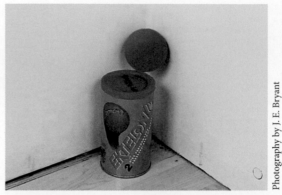

Photography by J. E. Bryant

PHOTO 11.10   Ball Hitting Ball Can: A Replay
Hinder.

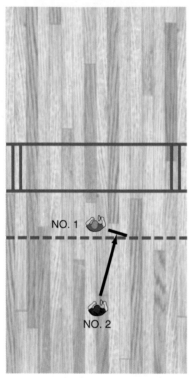

NO. 1

NO. 2

FIGURE 11.7   Being Hit by
Opponent's Shot: A Replay
Hinder.

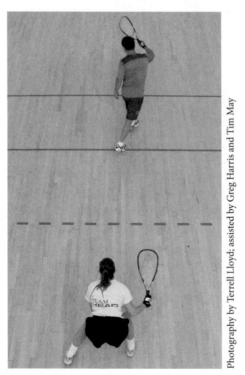

Photography by Terrell Lloyd; assisted by Greg Harris and Tim May

PHOTO 11.11   Screening the Ball: A
Replay Hinder.

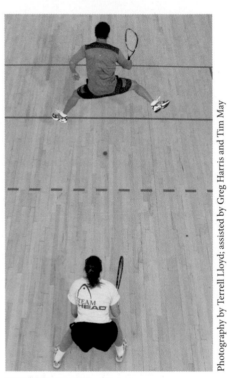

Photography by Terrell Lloyd; assisted by Greg Harris and Tim May

PHOTO 11.12   Straddle Ball: A
Replay hinder when screening the
opponent.

stroke believes the opponent's safety will be placed at risk.

The etiquette of calling a replay hinder rests initially with the player who creates the problem.

That player's obligation is to ask, "Do you want a hinder?" The response from the other player is either "Yes" or "No." If a hinder is identified by the offending player, the player restricted may say, "Hinder, please," and the opposing player has only the option of saying "Okay." In short, any request for a hinder is to be honored in an immediate affirmative manner. Hinders are to be requested immediately following the infraction so no question will arise concerning whether a hinder should be called.

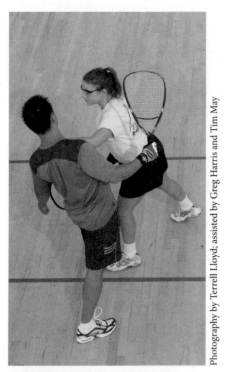

PHOTO 11.13 Two Players Colliding: A Replay Hinder.

A penalty hinder results in loss of a point to the opponent if the opponent was receiving and committed the infraction, and a sideout if the server committed the infraction.

A replay hinder requires a replay of the point. In a "friendly" game, penalty hinders should seldom happen, as the idea of the game is to play for enjoyment and fitness. If a player does resort to committing penalty hinders in that environment, a judicious response is not to play that person again.

Miscellaneous Rules

Rules include specific ones for use of the racquet. Often, beginners are not aware that the racquet must be held in one hand and remain in that hand throughout any rally. The racquet also must be attached to the wrist by the tether to reduce the possibility of injury. Another rule that is common knowledge but is often misunderstood is that the ball always must be struck only by the racquet for a legal return. Other commonly misunderstood rules include the following:

1. The ball must be dry before being placed in play.

2. A server may not take a running stride to execute the serve.

3. A receiver of serve may not cross the receiving line and move into the safety zone until the served ball has crossed the short line, thus eliminating a potentially hazardous situation (see Figure 11.8 and Photo 11.14).

4. A crotch shot strikes the crotch of the front wall and floor, ceiling, or side wall simultaneously.

5. During a serve, a crotch shot off the front wall is an out serve. A crotch-shot serve that strikes off the floor and back wall, or the side wall and floor beyond the short line is in play. During play, a crotch shot is always in play unless it hits the front wall.

6. Only the server is permitted to score after a winning rally.

Understanding the common rules of serving, hinders, and

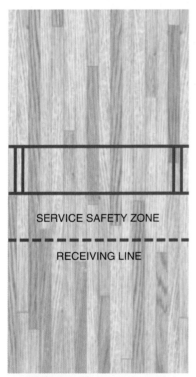

FIGURE 11.8 Five-foot Safety Zone.

SERVICE SAFETY ZONE

RECEIVING LINE

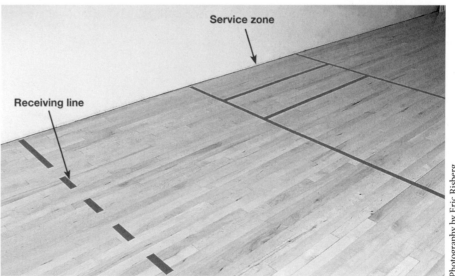

Service zone

Receiving line

PHOTO 11.14 Receiving Line in Relation to Service Zone.

scoring allows the novice the freedom to play the game early in skill development.

Beyond the Singles Game

The emphasis throughout this book has been on singles play. It is the safest form of racquetball, as there are just two players within an 800-square-foot area enclosed by four walls. Two additional games are played with regularity in a four-wall court area. One is **doubles**, a competition between two-player teams.

The other game, with three players, is called **cut-throat**.

Doubles

Rules that relate to doubles are distinct in some ways, including serving order, player hitting order, position during serve, and hinder situations. The serve order follows a sequence of one partner serving consecutive points until a sideout occurs, and then the second partner serving in a similar fashion until there is a second sideout.

The service order of the partners has one exception, and that fits only the first serving team: The first partner serves to the conclusion of serve, then the team exchanges with the receiving team. When the first serving team returns for the second round of serves, the first serving partner again begins serve, followed by the normal sequence of partner serve rotation.

The player hitting order, once the ball is placed in play by a serve, is the same as in the singles game, with team A hitting a serve, team B returning the serve, team A responding to return of serve, etc. Either player on a team may hit for that team in the rally.

During a serve, the serving team stands within the service zone as in singles play. One partner serves, and the other partner stands in the service box with his her back to the side wall, or a foot fault is called (see Photo 11.15).

If the partner in the doubles box is struck by the partner's serve, the serve is declared dead and the serve is executed again. Once the ball is in play, any ball that is hit by one partner and strikes the other partner is deemed a sideout or a handout if committed by the serving team, or a point for the serving team if committed by the receiving team.

The receiving team must stand behind the receiving line to receive serve. Hinders are the same as in singles play, but the possibility for hinder calls is magnified by the presence of four players on the court at one time.

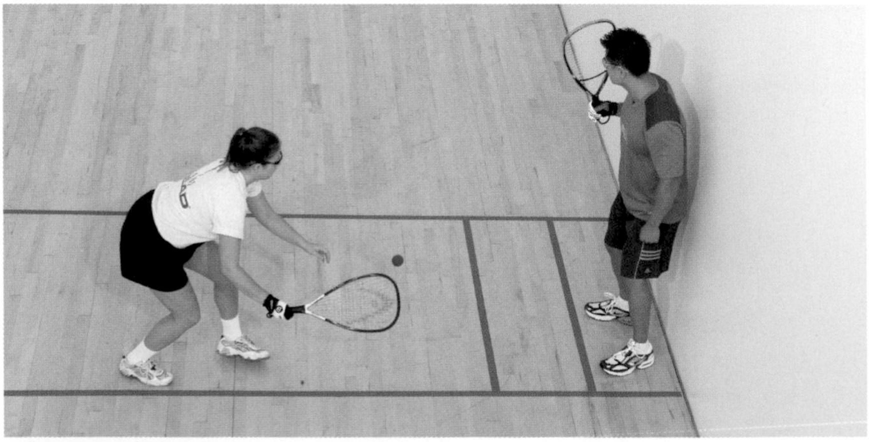

PHOTO 11.15   Doubles Serving Position.

Photography by Terrell Lloyd; assisted by Greg Harris and Tim May

Doubles Strategy

Because of the number of players on the court during a game of doubles, there is more risk for injury than when playing a single opponent.

Consequently, with four players on a small court at the same time, all players must *think* during play! Running into an opponent or your partner, striking another player instead of the ball, and, going for the same shot as another player will occur when players consider only the ball

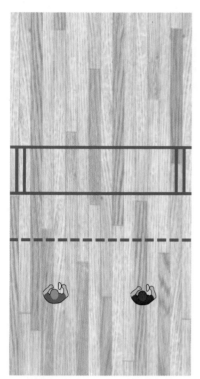

FIGURE 11.9 Playing Side by side.

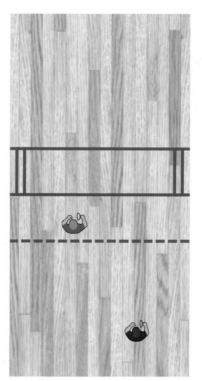

FIGURE 11.10 Up-and-Back Coverage.

and not the other participants on the court. Thus, to play doubles successfully, you must *think* while you play and communicate with your partner about playing strategy as well.

The first decision you and your partner must make is how you will work together to cover the court.

There are three basic ways to share court responsibility. The first, and most basic, is simply to divide the court in half lengthwise and play *side by side*. One player will take all balls landing on the right side of the court (see Figure 11.9), and his or her partner takes balls landing on the left side of the court. In this court strategy, each player must cover his or her side of the court regardless of where the ball touches the floor in relation to the front wall.

The key to the successful use of this positioning is to (1) assign the best player to take backhand shots, and (2) predetermine who will take balls rebounding down the middle of the court. This prevents both players

from "courteously" allowing the partner to take the middle-court shot and ending up with neither player reacting to the ball.

If a team has both a right-handed and a left-handed player, make sure that the players set up on the court so their forehand strokes are toward the nearest wall. The player with the best backhand then should be assigned to take balls that rebound down the middle of the court.

This position strategy is good for beginning players and for players who are approximately equal in playing ability. It allows each player to focus on a well-defined area of the court and concentrate on hitting the ball. This strategy also minimizes spontaneous decision-making and conflict between partners.

The second court position strategy is again to divide the court in half, but this time to identify a front-court and a back-court coverage, commonly referred to as *up-and-back* (see Figure 11.10).

In this strategy, one partner is positioned by the short line and the other is an arm's length from the back wall. Both players cover their area of the court from side wall to side wall.

This strategy is good for players who bring different playing strengths to the court. In particular, if one player is skilled in offensive kill shots, he or she should be the "up" player. If a player is particularly good at hitting defensive shots or taking shots that rebound off the back corners of the court, he or she should cover the back position.

Another way to decide who plays "up" is based on speed of movement. Good front-court play is best accomplished by players who are quick and agile. This is because the front player has to respond to opponents' kill shots from this position, and when receiving the serve, must readjust quickly from a service-return court position (back-court) to the service-court area.

If neither player has these qualities, an up-and-back strategy of court coverage is not advised. If both players have equal strength in both offensive and defensive returns and movement on the court, they can alternate the "up" and "back" positions. This can be done simply by predetermining that the partner not returning the serve will move to a forward-court position. The partner returning the serve will protect the back-court area.

The third strategy for court coverage, called *diagonal court coverage*, divides the court into two triangles. The triangles are determined by a diagonal boundary extending from the short line/side wall intersection to the opposite side wall/back wall juncture. Whether the diagonal is "drawn" toward the back right or left corner of the court depends on the partners' preference (see Figure 11.11), and which partner wants to cover the front- versus the back-court area. The fastest (offensive) player should cover the short line and very little of the back court. The defensive player should defend the back-court area and balls that rebound along the side wall within his or her triangle.

Again, the two partners must confer to determine who will play balls rebounding along the diagonal.

Make this decision before starting play! The side wall that each player "protects" is determined in the same way as the side-by-side strategy.

Keep the player with the strongest backhand on the left side of the court or, in the case of a right-handed/left-handed pairing, place the players' forehands toward the nearest wall.

This strategy should be used for players who are more experienced with the game, as it requires awareness of where balls will rebound to determine which partner should take the shot. It also can be effective for players of significantly different skill levels, with the more highly skilled player covering the front position along with the back corner and the less skilled player taking primarily defensive shots along the back wall.

In doubles it is important to find the weakness of the other team and play to that weakness. If the opposing team is in a *side-by-side alignment* and lacks the ability to return shots hit to the backhand, hitting to the backhand is an obvious strategy.

In addition, hitting the ball down the middle when opponents are playing this alignment often results in miscommunication and mishits.

A team that plays an *up-and-back alignment* should have an offensive strategy of gaining control of the center court and dominating play from that position. Hitting passing shots or ceiling shots past opponents playing this alignment reduces that team's effectiveness.

Doubles strategy requires control of the center court and the ability

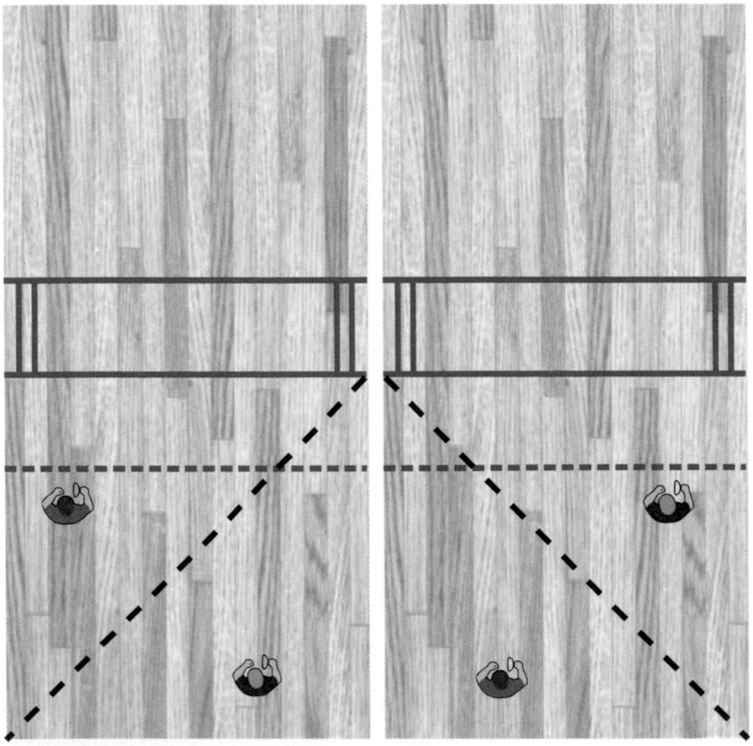

FIGURE 11.11   Diagonal Court Coverage.

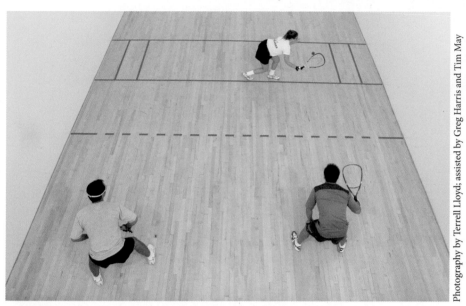

PHOTO 11.16   Cutthroat Serving Position.

Photography by Terrell Lloyd; assisted by Greg Harris and Tim May

to hit shots that eventually will put the opposing team out of position. Once out of position, the idea is to place a shot that neither doubles opponent can reach or return with any authority.

Generally, doubles play requires a defensive strategy. Hitting around-the-wall, ceiling, and passing shots keeps a beginning doubles team opponent off balance. Chasing shots heightens the risk for an error by a doubles team, resulting in a set-up kill shot by the opponents.

Working cooperatively and communicating are prime requirements for a successful doubles team. Keeping the opposing team off balance, covering for each other during a rally, and maintaining good court balance while controlling the center of the court are prerequisites for success.

Cut-throat

The **cut-throat** game is an unofficial racquetball game. There are basically two types of games to play. One cutthroat game is a two-against-one setup, with the receiving team playing as a doubles team and the serving player competing against that team. Following each sideout, the doubles team membership changes and the server becomes a part of a new doubles team. All play on the part of the doubles team as related to movement and position utilizes doubles rules, and all other play commences as in singles (see Photo 11.16 and Figure 11.12).

The second type of cut-throat game is a safer version and becomes a singles match with three players. One player is always sitting out a particular point by standing in a back-wall area while the other two players are playing. At the conclusion of each point, the noncompeting player enters the game as a receiver of the serve, and the player who lost the point steps out. If the server loses the point, the former receiver becomes the server. If the receiver loses the point, the server remains as server and play continues.

In both games of cut-throat, each player keeps an individual score, and the winner is the first player to gain 15 points. The game of cut-throat provides for a change-of-pace situation that permits three people to enjoy a game designed for two or four.

Cut-Throat Strategy

Cut-throat for the beginning player has its own strategy. Both types of cut-throat require the basic strategy of maintaining control of center court. Two-against-one cut-throat requires a combined doubles and singles strategy. Cut-throat played with one player sitting out is no more than a *singles match* scored as a cut-throat competition involving three players. Singles strategy applies to this game, and you are reminded to review Chapters 8 and 9.

Playing in a *two-against-one* set up requires a unique strategy because it is doubles against singles competition. The doubles team has the advantage of outnumbering the singles player,

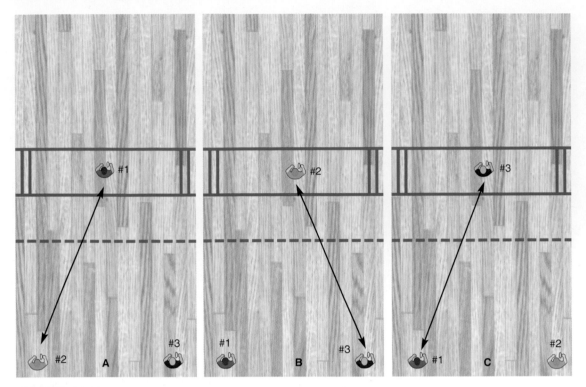

FIGURE 11.12   Serving Rotation Sequence for Cut-throat Game.

which means that the team can cover more court area and, with some skill, move the opposing singles player. The singles player has the advantage of being the server and, with a good serve, can place the doubles team at an immediate disadvantage. A good serve requires accurate placement, low drives with good velocity, and the shrewdness to force the doubles team out of position during a rally.

The doubles team has to assume a teamwork stance immediately. Remember that after each rotation, the team makeup changes. Keep in mind that each player is competing separately and yet is expected to function as a teammate when playing in a doubles configuration.

When returning serve, the doubles team has to concentrate on effective means of returning serve. Ceiling shots, although defensive, drive the singles player to the back wall, forcing the player to give up center-court control. Returning serve with a passing shot is also a good strategy,

because that type of shot also moves the singles player to the back court.

Once the singles player is on the defensive, the doubles team has the advantage.

The team should work hard at maintaining control of the center court, forcing the singles player to chase the ball to return it. Obviously, creating a situation that sets up a point-ending kill shot is a purposeful goal for the doubles team. Typically, that happens when the singles player is forced out of the center court, having been forced to move and chase the ball.

When playing the doubles position, communication is important. The two players have to talk and support each other while aggressively attacking the singles player.

The singles player must serve well to have a chance. Most cutthroat matches, as friendly competition, are played with the expectation that the server will alternate serves so that after each point the nonreceiving doubles partner of the previous point receives the next serve.

If this is the way the game is elected to be played, the singles player has to determine the weakness of the receiving double player to try to serve to that disadvantage. The goal of the serve has to be to force a weak return that allows the singles player to maintain control of the center court.

If a serve rotation mentioned above is not in effect, the singles player has the advantage of serving continuously to the weakest doubles partner. An alternative to attacking the weakest server is to serve down the middle of the court, creating the possibility of indecision on the part of the doubles team.

Once in a rally, the singles player does not have the luxury of sustaining play. It is important to execute winning shots, which means hitting a kill shot when it is set up, driving a passing shot low to the back corner of the doubles team, and hitting hard drive shots that force the doubles team to chase the ball. If the doubles team gains control of the center court, hitting to the back wall becomes critical for the singles player. A high side-wall pass shot works well in moving the team and allowing the singles player to regain control of the center area.

The serving rotation follows a sequence of server number one exchanging with the number-two player, who is a receiver. When the next sideout occurs, the number-two player, who has been the server, exchanges with the number-three player, who is the second receiver.

The sequence follows an exchange of the number-three player (who is the server) on the next sideout with the number-one player, who has moved through the sequence as receiver. Then the process is repeated (see Figures 11.12A–C).

This type of exchange alternates the receiver's position each time through the full serving sequence. If the number-two receiver started from a left-side receiving position during the first sequence, that number-two player would receive from the right side during the second sequence of return of serve.

Three-wall and One-wall Racquetball

Racquetball can be played on other surfaces and configurations. Three-wall and one-wall games have developed in city parks and school playgrounds, and sometimes are found on college campuses where the weather is warm enough to provide for year-round play.

Three-wall racquetball follows the same rules as the four-wall game. Scoring, serving, ball in play, hinders, and all other general rules are the same. Exceptions to this are the result of the court structure itself, which does not have a back wall or a ceiling, and typically has a side wall that does

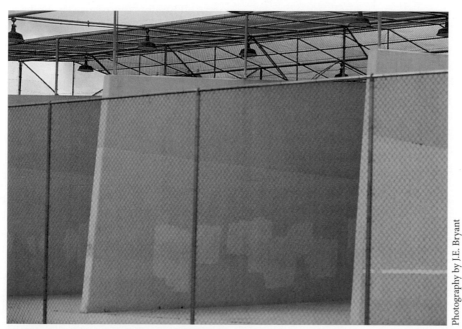

PHOTO 11.17 Three-wall Racquetball Courts.

Photography by J.E. Bryant

not extend completely to the long line (see Photo 11.17).

These exceptions are as follows:

- A ball in play that lands outside the long line (where the back wall normally would be) is a point or sideout (or handout), depending on the situation.
- A served ball that lands outside the long line is a fault serve (long), just as in four-wall if the ball strikes the back wall on the fly.
- In the three-wall courts, where the side walls extend only partially to the long line, a serve or a ball in play hit wide of the side line is considered a wide ball and is a point or sideout (handout), depending on the situation.
- A ball in play or a served ball that is hit above the front wall (there is often a screen that catches the ball so players are not continually chasing the ball) is considered a point or a sideout (handout).
- When the side wall does not extend fully to the long line, a replay hinder is called when a ball or player from an adjacent court crosses into a court with the ball in play.

One-wall racquetball also is similar to the four-wall game. Obviously, the major difference is that the one-wall game has only two playing surfaces: front wall and floor. The floor measures 20 feet wide and 34 feet long to the back edge of what is called the long line. The back edge of the short line is 16 feet from the front wall, and the service zone consists all of the space between the short line and the front wall.

With the exception of the court configuration, the game is played much as the four-wall game is played. Strategy is simplified to a power game, as there are no rebound angles to play off side walls or ceiling.

Sportsmanship Ethic

Racquetball has a sportsmanship ethic implying that the game is played for exercise and enjoyment. Coupled with that implication is the reality that most matches are played without officiating, so it is imperative to call each point or shot fairly and without prejudice. It is doubly important to recognize that no point is worth winning if you or your opponent are put at risk of injury.

The best example of the application of sportsmanship is the hinder, as many hinders have the potential for creating circumstances that could result in injury. The hinder call allows for players to consider the safety of their opponent and encourages a sportsmanship gesture because players call hinders on themselves and are expected to willingly accept hinder calls by their opponent.

The sportsmanship attitude extends to shaking hands following a match and being a good loser or a humble winner. The concept of sportsmanship is so much rhetoric in many other sports, but in racquetball, sportsmanship is a necessity.

POINTS to REMEMBER

When you warm up prior to playing, be sure to share the court in a side-by-side format.

A match consists of two 15-point games followed by a third game of 11 points if a tiebreaker is needed, and each game requires a one-point margin to win.

Common fault serves include "short," "three-wall," and "long" serves, resulting in a sideout if served in succession.

An out serve occurs in numerous situations, such as the ball not initially striking the front wall, and is penalized by loss of serve.

A replay hinder occurs as a result of unintentional action and requires replay of a rally.

A penalty hinder usually occurs when one player intentionally or unintentionally creates an action that impedes the opponent, resulting in loss of the rally.

A replay hinder is reflective of an unavoidable movement or action of a player that restricts the opponent from a fair chance to hit the ball, which then requires a replay of the point.

Sportsmanship is required in racquetball for safety purposes, and also because most matches are played on the honor system.

CHECKPOINTS

Answers are located on page 141.

1. A penalty hinder occurs when:
   a. a player refuses to move out of the way of an opponent's shot opportunity.
   b. player A hits player B with a shot to the front wall.
   c. a ball is hit between the legs of players A so player B is screened off from seeing the ball.
   d. a shot strikes an irregular spot on the court.

2. A replay hinder occurs when:
   a. player A gets too close to player B's shot attempt.
   b. player A shoves player B in order to reach the ball to return a shot.
   c. player A, on purpose, moves in front of player B's shot to the front wall.
   d. player A hits player B with a shot attempt to the front wall.

3. The two cut-throat games are:
   a. two-against-one with the serving team as a doubles pairing.
   b. two-against-one with the receiving team as a doubles pairing.
   c. singles play with the third player inactive.

   d. singles play with two players inactive.

4. Of the three strategic alignments in doubles, the alignment that reflects equal skill on the part of both players is:
   a. side-by-side.
   b. one up, one back.
   c. combination with the left side player covering two-thirds of the back court and one-half of the front court.
   d. combination with the right-side player covering one-third of the back court and one-half of the front court.

5. The most impacting strategy in doubles is for a team to:
   a. gain control of the center court.
   b. hit kill shots.
   c. hit drive passing shots.
   d. hit defensive shots.

6. In cut-throat, it is critical from a strategy standpoint for the singles player to:
   a. execute a winning shot as quickly as possible.
   b. hit high lobs to the corners when in control of the center court.

   c. go for a kill shot to end the rally when playing back.
   d. hit drives down the center of the court when in a rally.

7. Proper etiquette (and safety) requires that when returning a ball to an opponent, it is returned by:
   a. gently tossing the ball.
   b. throwing the ball.
   c. throwing on one bounce.
   d. rolling the ball.

8. The sportsmanship ethic in racquetball is essential. It is most related to all except one of the following:
   a. The game is played first and foremost for exercise and enjoyment.
   b. Most matches are played without an official, thus requiring honest calls on the part of all players.
   c. Safety is of major concern, and thus requires that hinders be called quickly and fairly to avoid excessive physical contact.
   d. The goal is to win at all costs, short of serious injury to the opposing player.

Appendix

Official Rules of Racquetball

Rules Notice

2007 USAR Official Rules of Racquetball
Includes Rule Changes Effective September 1, 2007. This updated rulebook contains several additions/revisions from the previously published version (©2004). The most significant changes affected Rule 2.4(e); Rule 3.9(j); Rule 3.17(a)6; Policy A.6; and Policy A.8.

Copyright Notice

Contents

1.0—The Game

1.1—Types Of Games

Racquetball is played by two or four players. When played by two, it is called singles and when played by four, doubles. A nontournament variation of the game that is played by three players is called cutthroat.

1.2—Description

Racquetball is a competitive game in which each player uses a strung racquet to serve and return the ball.

1.3—Objective

The objective is to win each rally by serving or re-turning the ball so the opponent is unable to keep the ball in play. A rally is over when a player (or team in doubles) is unable to hit the ball before it touches the floor twice, is unable to return the ball in such a manner that it touches the front wall before it touches the floor, or when a hinder is called.

1.4—Points and Outs

Points are scored only by the serving side when it serves an irretrievable serve (an ace) or wins a rally. Losing the serve is called a sideout in singles. In doubles, when the first server loses the serve, it is called a handout, and when the second server loses the serve, it is a sideout.

1.5—Match, Game, Tiebreaker

A match is won by the first side winning two games. The first 2 games of a match are played to 15 points. If each side wins 1 game, a tiebreaker game is played to 11 points.

2.0—Courts and Equipment

2.1—Court and Specifications

The specifications for the standard four-wall racquetball court are:

(a) Dimensions. The dimensions shall be 20 feet wide, 40 feet long and 20 feet high, with a back wall at least 12 feet high. All surfaces shall be in play, with the exception of any gallery opening, surfaces designated as out-of-play for a valid reason (such as being of a very different material or not in alignment with the back wall), and designated court hinders.

(b) Markings. Racquetball courts shall be marked with lines 1 1/2 inches wide as follows:

1. Short Line. The back edge of the short line is midway between, and is parallel with, the front and back walls.

2. Service Line. The front edge of the service line is parallel with, and five feet in front of, the back edge of the short line.

3. Service Zone. The service zone is the 5' x 20' area bounded by the bottom edges of the side walls and by the outer edges of the short line and the service line.

4. Service Boxes. The service boxes, used in doubles play, are located at each end of the service zone and are designated by lines parallel with the side walls [see 4.2(b)]. The edge of the line nearest to the center of the court shall be 18 inches from the nearest side wall.

5. Drive Serve Lines. The drive serve lines, which form the drive serve zones, are parallel with the side wall and are within the service zone. For each line, the edge of the line nearest to the center of the court shall be three feet from the nearest side wall.

6. Receiving Line. The receiving line is a broken line parallel to the short line. The back edge of the receiving line is five feet from the back edge of the short line. The receiving line begins with a line 21 inches long that extends from each side wall. These lines are connected by an alternate series of six-inch spaces and six-inch lines. This will result in a line composed of 17 six-inch spaces, 16 six-inch lines, and 2 twenty-one-inch lines.

7. Safety Zone. The safety zone is the 5' x 20' area bounded by the bottom edges of the side walls and by the back edges of the short line and the receiving line. The zone is observed only during the serve. See Rules 3.10(i) and 3.11(a).

2.2—Ball Specifications

(a) The standard racquetball shall be 2 1/4 inches in diameter; weigh approximately 1.4 ounces; have a hardness of 55–60 inches durometer; and bounce 68–72 inches from a 100-inch drop at a temperature of 70–74 degrees Fahrenheit.

(b) Only a ball having the approval of the USAR may be used in a USAR-sanctioned tournament.

2.3—Ball Selection

(a) A ball shall be selected by the referee for use in each match. During the match the referee may, based on personal discretion or at the request of a player or team, replace the ball. Balls that are not round or which bounce erratically shall not be used.

(b) If possible, the referee and players should agree to an alternate ball, so that in the event of breakage, the second ball can be put into play immediately.

2.4—Racquet Specifications

(a) The racquet, including bumper guard and all solid parts of the handle, may not exceed 22 inches in length.

(b) The racquet frame may be any material judged safe.

(c) The racquet frame must include a cord that must be securely attached to the player's wrist.

(d) The string of the racquet must be gut, monofilament, nylon, graphite, plastic, metal, or a combination thereof, and must not mark or deface the ball.

(e) Using an illegal racquet will result in forfeiture of the game in progress or, if discovered between games, forfeiture of the preceding game. The penalty for playing with an otherwise legal racquet with a grip extending beyond the 22-inch limit if noted during the course of a game shall be a technical foul and a timeout to correct the problem. Subsequent violations will result in the loss of the game in process. If the challenged racquet is found to be within the 22-inch limit, then a timeout will be charged to the player who made the challenge.

2.5—Apparel

(a) All players must wear lensed eyewear that has been warranted by its manufacturer or distributor as (1) designed for use in racquetball and (2) meeting or exceeding the then-current and full ASTM F803 standard. This rule applies to all persons, including those who wear corrective lenses. The eyewear must be unaltered and worn as designed at all times. A player who fails to wear proper eyewear will be assessed a technical foul and a timeout to obtain proper eyewear [see Rule 3.17(a)(9)]. A second infraction in the same match will result in immediate forfeiture of the match.

Certifications & Compliance. The USAR maintains a reference list of eyewear so warranted by their manufacturers, and provides that list to each sanctioned event (an eyewear list dated more than 90 days prior to the first day of the tournament will be deemed invalid for the purpose of determining compliance with this eyewear rule). In addition, the list is available online at the USAR.org website (indexed under "eyeguards"), and individual copies may be requested by calling the USAR National Office at (719) 635-5396.

To be used in sanctioned competition, protective eyewear must:

- bear a permanent, physical stamp of the appropriate "ASTM-F803" citation on the frame itself
- appear on the ASTM reference listing
- bear the "Protective Eyewear Certification Council" [PECC] seal of approval for the ASTM standard
- be certified in writing by the maker that it complies with the required ASTM standard (in this instance, the player must be able to provide written, adequate proof—on demand—at any sanctioned event, before such eyewear may be used).

(b) Clothing and Shoes. The clothing may be of any color; however, a player may be required to change wet, extremely loose-fitting, or otherwise distracting garments. Insignias and writing on the clothing must be considered to be in good taste by the tournament director. Shoes must have soles which do not mark or damage the floor.

(c) Equipment Requirements During Warm-up. Proper eyeguards [see 2.5(a)] must be worn and wrist cords must be used during any on-court warm-up period. The referee should give a technical warning to any person who fails to comply and assess a technical foul if that player continues to not comply after receiving such a warning.

3.0—Play Regulations

3.1—Serve
In Open Division competition, the server will have one opportunity to put the ball into play [see Section 5.0 for complete, one-serve modifications]. In all other divisions, the server will have two opportunities to put the ball into play. The player or team winning the coin toss has the option to either serve or receive at the start of the first game. The second game will begin in reverse order of the first game. The player or team scoring the highest total of points in games 1 and 2 will have the option to serve or receive first at the start of the tiebreaker. If both players or teams score an equal number of points in the first two games, another coin toss will take place and the winner of the toss will have the option to serve or receive.

3.2—Start
The server may not start the service motion until the referee has called the score or "second serve." The referee shall call the score as both server and receiver prepare to return to their respective positions, shortly after the previous rally has ended—even if the players are not ready. The serve is started from any place within the service zone. (Certain drive serves are an exception. See Rule 3.6.) Neither the ball nor any part of either foot may extend beyond either line of the service zone when initiating the service motion. Stepping on, but not beyond, the lines is permitted. However, when completing the service motion, the server may step beyond the service (front) line provided that some part of both feet remain on or inside the line until the served ball passes the short line. The server may not step beyond the short line until the ball passes the short line. See Rule 3.9(a) and 3.10(i) for penalties for violations.

3.3—Manner
After taking a set position inside the service zone, a player may begin the service motion—any continuous movement that results in the ball being served. Once the service motion begins, when the ball leaves the hand, it must next bounce on the floor in the zone and then, without touching anything else, be struck by the racquet before it bounces on the floor a second time. After being struck, the ball must hit the front wall first and on the rebound hit the floor beyond the back edge of the short line, either with or without touching one of the side walls.

3.4—Readiness
The service motion shall not begin until the referee has called the score or "second serve" and the server has visually checked the receiver's readiness.

3.5—Delays

Except as noted in Rule 3.5(b), the referee may call a technical foul for delays exceeding 10 seconds.

(a) The 10-second rule applies to the server and receiver simultaneously. Concurrently, they are allowed up to 10 seconds after the score is called to serve or be ready to receive. It is the server's responsibility to look and be certain the receiver is ready. If a receiver is not ready, they must signal by raising the racquet above the head or completely turning the back to the server. (These are the only two acceptable signals.)

(b) Serving while the receiving player/team is signaling "not ready" is a fault serve.

(c) After the score is called, if the server looks at the receiver and the receiver is not signaling "not ready," the server may then serve. If the receiver attempts to signal "not ready" after that point, the signal shall not be acknowledged and the serve becomes legal.

3.6—Drive Service Zones

There is a drive serve line three feet from each side wall in the service zone. Viewed one at a time, each drive serve line divides the service zone into a 3-foot and a 17-foot section. The player may drive serve between the body and the side wall nearest to where the service motion began only if the player, the racquet, and ball (until it is struck) starts and remains outside of that 3-foot drive service zone until the served ball crosses the short line. A drive serve involving "any continuous movement" (see Rule 3.3—Manner), beginning in one 3-foot drive service zone and continuing into the opposite 3-foot drive service zone, is a fault serve.

(a) The drive serve zones are not observed for cross-court drive serves, the hard-Z, soft-Z, lob, or half-lob serves.

(b) The 3-foot line is part of the 3-foot zone and defines a plane that, if broken, is an infraction [see Rule 3.9(g)].

3.7—Defective Serves

Defective serves are of three types resulting in penalties as follows:

(a) Dead-ball Serve. A dead-ball serve results in no penalty and the server is given another serve (without canceling a prior fault serve).

(b) Fault Serve. Two fault serves result in an out (either a sideout or a handout).

(c) Out Serve. An out serve results in an out (either a sideout or a handout).

3.8—Dead-ball Serves

Dead-ball serves do not cancel any previous fault serve. The following are dead-ball serves:

(a) Court Hinders. A serve that takes an irregular bounce because it hit a wet spot or an irregular surface on the court is a dead-ball serve. In addition, any serve that hits any surface designated by local rules as an obstruction rather than being out-of-play.

(b) Broken Ball. If the ball is determined to have broken on the serve, a new ball shall be substituted and the serve shall be replayed, not canceling any prior fault serve.

3.9—Fault Serves

The following serves are faults and any two in succession result in an out:

(a) Foot Faults. A foot fault results when:

1. At the start of or during the service motion, any part of the server (or doubles partner), including the racquet, touches the floor outside of the service zone.

2. At the end of the serve, the server steps with either foot on the floor beyond the service line (with no part of the foot on the line or inside the service zone) before the served ball crosses the short line.

(b) Short Service. A short serve is any served ball that first hits the front wall and, on the rebound, hits the floor on or in front of the short line either with or without touching a side wall.

(c) Three-wall Serve. A three-wall serve is any served ball that first hits the front wall and, on the rebound, strikes both side walls before touching the floor.

(d) Ceiling Serve. A ceiling serve is any served ball that first hits the front wall and then touches the ceiling (with or without touching a side wall).

(e) Long Serve. A long serve is a served ball that first hits the front wall and rebounds to the back wall before touching the floor (with or without touching a side wall).

(f) Bouncing Ball Outside Service Zone. Bouncing the ball outside the service zone, including the ball touching a side wall, as a part of the service motion is a fault serve.

(g) Illegal Drive Serve. A drive serve in which the player fails to observe the 17-foot drive service zone outlined in Rule 3.6.

(h) Screen Serve. A served ball that first hits the front wall and on the rebound passes so closely to the server, or server's partner in doubles, that it prevents the receiver from having a clear view of the ball. (The receiver is obligated to take up good court position, near center court, to obtain that view.)

(i) In one-serve play, if a serve is called a screen, the server will be allowed one more opportunity to hit a legal serve. Two consecutive screen serves result in an out.

(j) Serving Before the Receiver is Ready. A serve is made while the receiver is not ready as described in Rule 3.5(b). In one-serve play, if a serve is made while the receiver is not ready as described in Rule 3.5(b), the server will be allowed one more opportunity to hit a legal serve.

3.10—Out Serves
Any of the following results in an out:

(a) Two Consecutive Fault Serves [see Rule 3.9], or a single fault serve in one-serve play [see exceptions: 5.0].

(b) Missed Serve Attempt. Any attempt to strike the ball that results in a total miss or in the ball touching any part of the server's body, including the foot. Also, allowing the ball to bounce more than once during the service motion.

(c) Touched Serve. Any served ball that on the rebound from the front wall touches the server or server's racquet before touching the floor, or any ball intentionally stopped or caught by the server or server's partner.

(d) Fake or Balk Serve. Any movement of the racquet toward the ball during the serve that is noncontinuous and done for the purpose of deceiving the receiver. If a balk serve occurs, but the referee believes that no deceit was involved, the option of declaring "no serve" and having the serve replayed without penalty can be exercised.

(e) Illegal Hit. An illegal hit includes contacting the ball twice, carrying the ball, or hitting the ball with the handle of the racquet or part of the body or uniform.

(f) Non-front Wall Serve. Any served ball that does not strike the front wall first.

(g Crotch Serve. Any served ball that hits the crotch of the front wall and floor, front wall and side wall, or front wall and ceiling is an out serve (because it did not hit the front wall first). A serve into the crotch of the back wall and floor is a good serve and in play. A served ball that hits the crotch of the side wall and floor beyond the short line is in play.

(h) Out-of-Court Serve. An out-of-court serve is any served ball that first hits the front wall and, before striking the floor, either goes out of the court or hits a surface above the normal playing area of the court that has been declared as out-of-play for a valid reason [See Rule 2.1(a)].

(i) Safety Zone Violation. An immediate loss of serve shall result if, after the serve has been struck, the server or doubles partner steps into the safety zone before the served ball passes the short line.

3.11—Return of Serve
(a) Receiving Position
1. The receiver may not break the plane of the receiving line with the racquet or body until the ball either bounces in the safety zone or else crosses the receiving line. For example, if the receiver steps on the dashed receiving line with either foot (with any part of the foot contacting the line), a point shall be called for the server.
2. The follow-through may carry the receiver or the racquet past the receiving line, but neither may break the plane of the short line unless the ball is struck after rebounding off the back wall.
3. Any violation by the receiver results in a point for the server.

(b) Defective Serve. A player on the receiving side may not intentionally catch or touch a served ball (such as an apparently long or short serve) until the referee has made a call or the ball has touched the floor for a second time. Violation results in a point.

(c) Legal Return. After a legal serve, a player receiving the serve must strike the ball on the fly or after the first bounce, and before the ball touches the floor the second time; and return the ball to the front wall, either directly or after touching one or both side walls, the back wall or the ceiling, or any combination of those surfaces. A returned ball must touch the front wall before touching the floor.

(d) Failure to Return. The failure to return a serve results in a point for the server.

(e) Other Provisions. Except as noted in this rule (3.11), the return of serve is subject to all provisions of Rules 3.13 through 3.15.

3.12—Changes of Serve
(a) Outs. A server is entitled to continue serving until one of the following occurs:
1. Out Serve. See Rule 3.10.
2. Two Consecutive Fault Serves [see Rule 3.9], or a single fault serve in one-serve play [see exceptions: 5.0].

3. Failure to Return Ball. Player or team fails to keep the ball in play as required by Rule 3.11(c).

4. Penalty Hinder. Player or team commits a penalty hinder which results in an out. See Rule 3.15.

(b) Sideout. Retiring the server in singles is called a sideout.

(c) Effect of Sideout. When the server (or serving team) receives a sideout, the server becomes the receiver and the receiver becomes the server.

3.13—Rallies

All of the play that occurs after the successful return of serve is called the rally. Play shall be conducted according to the following rules:

(a) Legal Hits. Only the head of the racquet may be used at any time to return the ball. The racquet may be held in one or both hands. Switching hands to hit a ball, touching the ball with any part of the body or uniform, or removing the wrist safety cord during a rally results in a loss of the rally.

(b) One Touch. The player or team trying to return the ball may touch or strike the ball only once or else the rally is lost. The ball may not be carried. (A carried ball is one that rests on the racquet long enough that the effect is more of a sling or throw than a hit.)

(c) Failure to Return. Any of the following constitutes a failure to make a legal return during a rally:

1. The ball bounces on the floor more than once before being hit.

2. The ball does not reach the front wall on the fly.

3. The ball is hit such that it goes into the gallery or wall opening or else hits a surface above the normal playing area of the court that has been declared as out-of-play [See Rule 2.1(a)].

4. A ball that obviously does not have the velocity or direction to hit the front wall strikes another player.

5. A ball struck by a player hits that player or that player's partner.

6. Committing a penalty hinder. See Rule 3.15.

7. Switching hands during a rally.

8. Failure to use a racquet wrist safety cord.

9. Touching the ball with the body or uniform.

10. Carrying or slinging the ball with the racquet.

(d) Effect of Failure to Return. Violations of Rules 3.13(a) through (c) result in a loss of rally. If the serving player or team loses the rally, it is an out.

If the receiver loses the rally, it results in a point for the server.

(e) Return Attempts. The ball remains in play until it touches the floor a second time, regardless of how many walls it makes contact with—including the front wall. If a player swings at the ball and misses it, the player may continue to attempt to return the ball until it touches the floor for the second time.

(f) Broken Ball. If there is any suspicion that a ball has broken during a rally, play shall continue until the end of the rally. The referee or any player may request the ball be examined. If the referee decides the ball is broken, the ball will be replaced and the rally replayed. The server resumes play at first serve. The only proper way to check for a broken ball is to squeeze it by hand. (Checking the ball by striking it with a racquet will not be considered a valid check and shall work to the disadvantage of the player or team that struck the ball after the rally.)

(g) Play Stoppage

1. If a foreign object enters the court, or any other outside interference occurs, the referee shall stop the play immediately and declare a replay hinder.

2. If a player loses any apparel, equipment, or other article, the referee shall stop play immediately and declare a penalty hinder or replay hinder as described in Rule 3.15(i).

(h) Replays. Whenever a rally is replayed for any reason, the server resumes play at first serve. A previous fault serve is not considered.

3.14—Replay Hinders

A rally is replayed without penalty and the server resumes play at first serve whenever a replay hinder occurs. Also, see Rule 3.15, which describes conditions under which a penalty hinder might be declared and result in loss of the rally.

(a) Situations

1. Court Hinders. The referee should stop play immediately whenever the ball hits any part of the court that was designated prior to the match as a court hinder (such as a vent grate). The referee should also stop play (i) when the ball takes an irregular bounce as a result of contacting an irregular surface (such as court light or vent) or after striking a wet spot on the floor or wall, and (ii) when, in the referee's opinion, the irregular bounce affected the rally.

2. Ball Hits Opponent. When an opponent is hit by a return shot in flight, it is a replay hinder. If the opponent is struck by a ball that obviously did not have the velocity or direction to reach the front wall, it is not a hinder, and the player who hit the ball will lose the rally. A player who has been hit by the ball can stop play and make the call, though the call must be made immediately and acknowledged by the referee. Note this interference may, under certain conditions, be declared a penalty hinder. See Rule 3.15.

3. Body Contact. If body contact occurs which the referee believes was sufficient to stop the rally, either for the purpose of preventing injury by further contact or because the contact prevented a player from being able to make a reasonable return, the referee shall call a hinder. Incidental body contact in which the offensive player clearly will have the advantage should not be called a hinder, unless the offensive player obviously stops play. Contact with the racquet on the follow-through normally is not considered a hinder for either player.

4. Screen Ball. Any ball rebounding from the front wall so close to the body of the defensive player that it prevents the offensive player from having a clear view of the ball. (The referee should be careful not to make the screen call so quickly that it takes away a good offensive opportunity.) A ball that passes between the legs of a player who has just returned the ball is not automatically a screen. It depends on whether the other player is impaired as a result. Generally, the call should work to the advantage of the offensive player.

5. Backswing Hinder. Any body or racquet contact, on the backswing or on the way to or just prior to returning the ball, which impairs the hitter's ability to take a reasonable swing. This call can be made by the player attempting the return, though the call must be made immediately and is subject to the referee's approval. Note the interference may be considered a penalty hinder. See Rule 3.15.

6. Safety Holdup. Any player about to execute a return, who believes that striking the opponent with the ball or racquet is likely, may immediately stop play and request a replay hinder. This call must be made immediately and is subject to acceptance and approval of the referee. (The referee will grant a replay hinder if it is believed the holdup was reasonable and the player would have been able to return the shot. The referee may also call a penalty hinder if warranted.)

7. Other Interference. Any other unintentional interference that prevents an opponent from having a fair chance to see or return the ball. Example: When a ball from another court enters the court during a rally or when a referee's call on an adjacent court obviously distracts a player.

(b) Effect of Hinders. The referee's call of hinder stops play and voids any situation that follows, such as the ball hitting the player. The only hinders that may be called by a player are described in Rules (2), (5), and (6) above, and all of these are subject to the approval of the referee. A replay hinder stops play and the rally is replayed. The server resumes play at first serve.

(c) Responsibility. While making an attempt to return the ball, a player is entitled to a fair chance to see and return the ball. It is the responsibility of the side that has just hit the ball to move so the receiving side may go straight to the ball and have an unobstructed view of and swing at the ball. However, the receiver is responsible for making a reasonable effort to move toward the ball and must have a reasonable chance to return the ball for any type of hinder to be called.

3.15—Penalty Hinders

A penalty hinder results in the loss of the rally. A penalty hinder does not necessarily have to be an intentional act. Replay hinders are described in Rule 3.14. Any of the following results in a penalty hinder:

(a) Failure to Move. A player does not move sufficiently to allow an opponent a shot straight to the front wall as well as a cross-court shot, which is a shot directly to the front wall at an angle that would cause the ball to rebound directly to the rear corner farthest from the player hitting the ball. In addition, when a player moves in such a direction that it prevents an opponent from taking either of these shots.

(b) Stroke Interference. This occurs when a player moves, or fails to move, so that the opponent returning the ball does not have a free, unimpeded swing. This includes unintentionally moving in a direction that prevents the opponent from making a shot.

(c) Blocking. Moves into a position which blocks the opponent from getting to, or returning, the ball; or in doubles, the offensive player who is not returning the ball hinders or impedes either defensive player's ability to move into a position to cover the pending shot that comes into play.

(d) Moving into the Ball. Moves in the way and is struck by the ball just played by the opponent.

(e) Pushing. Deliberately pushes or shoves opponent during a rally.

(f) Intentional Distractions. Deliberate shouting, stamping of feet, waving of racquet, or any other manner of disrupting one's opponent.

(g) View Obstruction. A player moves across an opponent's line of vision just before the opponent strikes the ball.

(h) Wetting the Ball. The players, particularly the server, should ensure that the ball is dry prior to the serve. Any wet ball that is not corrected prior to the serve shall result in a penalty hinder against the server.

(i) Apparel or Equipment Loss. If a player loses any apparel, equipment, or other article, play shall be immediately stopped and that player shall be called for a penalty hinder, unless the player has just hit a shot that could not be retrieved. If the loss of equipment is caused by a player's opponent, then a replay hinder should be called. If the opponent's action is judged to have been avoidable, then the opponent should be called for a penalty hinder.

3.16—Timeouts

(a) Rest Periods. Each player or team is entitled to three 30-second timeouts in games to 15 and two 30-second timeouts in games to 11. Timeouts may not be called by either side once the service motion has begun. Calling for a timeout when none remain or after the service motion has begun will result in the assessment of a technical foul for delay of game. If a player takes more than 30 seconds for a single timeout, the referee may automatically charge any remaining timeouts, as needed, for any extra time taken. Once all time allowed has expired, a delay-of-game technical foul can be assessed. A player who leaves the court should call a timeout or else advise the referee of the reason for leaving the court. If a player leaves the court without advising the referee, a timeout may be charged to that player. If none remain,

the referee may assess a technical foul for delay of game; however, the referee may excuse a delay if the player's reason for leaving was to correct a problem affecting the playability of the court, such as obtaining a towel to dry the court or disposing of some foreign material from the court.

(b) Injury. If a player is injured during the course of a match because of contact, such as with the ball, racquet, wall, floor, or another player, an injury timeout will be awarded. While a player may call more than one timeout for the same injury or for additional injuries that occur during the match, a player is not allowed more than a total of 15 minutes of rest for injury during the entire match. If the injured player is not able to resume play after total rest of 15 minutes, the match shall be awarded to the opponent. 1) Should any external bleeding occur, the referee must halt play as soon as the rally is over, charge an injury timeout to the person who is bleeding, and not allow the match to continue until the bleeding has stopped. 2) Muscle cramps and pulls, fatigue, and other ailments that are not caused by direct contact on the court will not be considered an injury. Injury time is also not allowed for preexisting conditions.

(c) Equipment Timeouts. Players are expected to keep all clothing and equipment in good, playable condition and are expected to use regular timeouts and time between games for adjustment and replacement of equipment. If a player or team is out of timeouts and the referee determines that an equipment change or adjustment is necessary for fair and safe continuation of the match, the referee may grant an equipment timeout not to exceed two minutes. The referee may allow additional time under unusual circumstances.

(d) Between Games. The rest period between the first two games of a match is two minutes. If a tiebreaker is necessary, the rest period between the second and third game is five minutes.

(e) Postponed Games. Any games postponed by referees shall be resumed with the same score as when postponed.

3.17—Technial Fouls and Warning

(a) Technical Fouls. The referee is empowered to deduct one point from a player's or team's score when, in the referee's sole judgment, the player is being overtly and deliberately abusive. If the player or team against whom the technical foul was assessed does not resume play immediately, the referee is empowered to forfeit the match in favor of the opponent. Some examples of actions that can result in technical fouls are:

1. Profanity.
2. Excessive arguing.
3. Threat of any nature to opponent or referee.
4. Excessive or hard striking of the ball between rallies.
5. Slamming of the racquet against walls or floor, slamming the door, or any action that might result in damage to the court or injury to other players.
6. Delay of game. Examples include (i) taking too much time to dry the court; (ii) excessive questioning of the referee about the rules; (iii) exceeding the time allotted for warm-up (see Policy A.8), timeouts, or between games; (iv) calling a timeout when none remain, or after the service motion begins; or (v) taking more than 10 seconds to serve or be ready to receive serve.
7. Intentional front-line foot fault to negate a bad lob serve.
8. Anything the referee considers unsportsmanlike behavior.
9. Failure to wear lensed eyewear designed for racquet sports [See Rule 2.5(a)] is an automatic technical foul on the first infraction, plus a mandatory timeout (to acquire the proper eyewear) will be charged against the offending player. A second infraction by that player during the match will result in automatic forfeiture of the match.

(b) Technical Warnings. If a player's behavior is not so severe as to warrant a technical foul, a technical warning may be issued without the deduction of a point.

(c) Effect of Technical Foul or Warning. If a referee issues a technical foul, one point shall be removed from the offender's score. No point will be deducted if a referee issues a technical warning. In either case, a technical foul or warning should be accompanied by a brief explanation. Issuing a technical foul or warning has no effect on who will be serving when play resumes. If a technical foul occurs when the offender has no points or between games, the result will be that the offender's score becomes minus one (-1).

4.0—Doubles

4.1—Doubles Team

(a) A doubles team shall consist of two players who meet either the age requirements or player classification requirements to participate in a particular division of play. A team with different skill levels must play in the division of the player with the higher level of ability. When playing in an adult age division, the team must play in the division of the younger player. When playing in a junior age division, the team must play in the division of the older player.

(b) A change in playing partners may be made so long as the first match of the posted team has not begun. For this purpose only, the match will be considered started once the teams have been called to the court. The team must notify the tournament director of the change prior to the beginning of the match.

4.2—Serve in Doubles

(a) Order of Serve. Before the match begins, each team shall inform the referee of their team's order of service, which shall be followed throughout the match. The order of serve may be changed between games, provided that the referee has been verbally notified before the first serve of the new game. At the beginning of each game, when the first server of the first team to serve is out, the team is out. Thereafter, both players on each team shall serve until the team receives a hand-out and a sideout.

(b) Partner's Position. On each serve, the server's partner shall stand erect with back to the side wall and with both feet on the floor within the service box from the moment the server begins the service motion until the served ball passes the short line. Violations are called foot faults. However, if the server's partner enters the safety zone before the ball passes the short line, the server loses service.

(c) Changes of Serve. In doubles, the side is retired when both partners have lost service, except that the team that serves first at the beginning of each game loses the serve when the first server is retired.

4.3—Fault Serve in Doubles

(a) The server's partner is not in the service box with both feet on the floor and back to (but not necessarily against) the side wall from the time the server begins the service motion until the ball passes the short line.

(b) A served ball that hits the doubles partner while in the doubles box results in a fault serve.

(c) In one-serve play, if a serve hits the nonserving partner while standing in the box, the server will be allowed one more opportunity to hit a legal serve. Hitting the nonserving partner twice results in an out.

(d) In one-serve play, consecutive faults—such as (i) a screen serve followed by hitting the nonserving partner or (ii) hitting the nonserving partner followed by serving while the receiver is not ready—results in an out.

4.4—Out Serve in Doubles

(a) Out-of-Order Serve. In doubles, when either partner serves out of order, the points scored by that server will be subtracted and an out serve will be called: if the second server serves out of order, the out serve will be applied to the first server and the second server will resume serving. If the player designated as the first server serves out of order, a sideout will be called. The referee should call "no serve" as soon as an out-of-order serve occurs. If no points are scored while the team is out of order, only the out penalty will have to be assessed. However, if points are scored before the out-of-order condition is noticed and the referee cannot recall the number, the referee may enlist the aid of the line judges (but not the crowd) to recall the number of points to be deducted.

(b) Ball Hits Partner. A served ball that hits the doubles partner while outside the doubles box results in loss of serve.

4.5—Return in Doubles

(a) The rally is lost if one player hits that same player's partner with an attempted return.

(b) If one player swings at the ball and misses it, both partners may make further attempts to return the ball until it touches the floor the second time. Both partners on a side are entitled to return the ball.

RULES MODIFICATION
5.0—One Serve

The USAR's standard rules governing racquetball play will be followed, but only one serve is allowed. Therefore, any fault serve is an out serve, with a few exceptions [noted separately below, and within the text rules cited]. [See Rule 3.9 FAULT SERVES (Screens).]

(i) In one-serve play, if a serve is called a screen, the server will be allowed one more opportunity

to hit a legal serve, except if the serve is also defective for some other reason, such as being long or short. Two consecutive screen serves result in an out. [See Rule 3.9(j) (Serving before the Receiver is Ready).]

(j) In one-serve play, if a serve is made while the receiver is not ready as described in Rule 3.5(b), the server will be allowed one more opportunity to hit a legal serve. [See Rule 4.3(c) (Serve hits partner).]

(c) In one-serve play, if a serve hits the nonserving partner while standing in the box, the server will be allowed one more opportunity to hit a legal serve. Hitting the nonserving partner twice results in an out. [Consecutive faults]

(d) In one-serve play, consecutive faults—either (i) a screen serve followed by hitting the nonserving partner or (ii) hitting the nonserving partner followed by a screen serve—results in an out.

6.0—Multi-bounce

6.1—Basic Return Rule

In general, the ball remains in play as long as it is bouncing. However, the player may swing only once at the ball, and the ball is considered dead at the point it stops bouncing and begins to roll. Also, anytime the ball rebounds off the back wall, it must be struck before it crosses the short line on the way to the front wall, except as explained in Rule 6.2.

6.2—Blast Rule

If the ball caroms from the front wall to the back wall on the fly, the player may hit the ball from any place on the court—including past the short line—so long as the ball is still bouncing.

6.3—Front Wall Lines

Two parallel lines (tape may be used) should be placed across the front wall such that the bottom edge of one line is three feet above the floor and the bottom edge of the other line is one foot above the floor. During the rally, any ball that hits the front wall (i) below the 3-foot line and (ii) either on or above the one-foot line must be returned before it bounces a third time. However, if the ball hits below the one-foot line, it must be returned before it bounces twice. If the ball hits on or above the three-foot line, the ball must be returned as described in the basic return rule.

6.4—Games and Matches

All games are played to 11 points, and the first side to win 2 games wins the match.

7.0—Outdoor Racquetball

7.1—Court Specifications

Outdoor courts vary in size, and there is no "official size." Generally, outdoor courts either have no or a very limited ceiling. They usually have no back walls; however, some courts may have a nonconnected back-wall surface considered part of the playing area. Outdoor courts can be classified as one of two general types:

(a) One-wall. A one-wall court has no side walls that do not extend more than a few feet.

(b) Three-wall. The front wall is usually at least 20 feet wide and at least 20 feet high. The side walls generally are at least 20 feet long and 20 feet high where they meet the front wall and are often tapered as they come toward the back court.

7.2—Court Markings

Generally, the markings are the same as the USAR's standard rules, except that on an outdoor court, there is no receiving (five-foot) line. Since the size of outdoor courts may vary, the exact placement of other lines may also vary. Both side lines and a back line are drawn, as needed, to denote a 20 foot-by-40-foot "in-play" area on the surface of the court. Some outdoor courts may also have singles service lines to reduce the server's advantage. These lines are usually placed 18 inches inside each side line and run from the short line to the back line. These lines are only in force during the serve and are not used for doubles play.

7.3—Apparel

Shirts are not required in the outdoor game.

7.4—Play Regulations

(a) All divisions follow the USAR's basic one-serve rules. Generally, a rally must be played for the receiver(s) to win a point or take possession of the serve.

(b) In doubles, the nonserving partner may take a position in the normal doubles box or outside the court beyond the back line or side line. If the nonserving partner hinders the receiving team on the return of serve, the referee may call a penalty hinder. In one-wall, the nonserving partner may not step onto the playing zone of the court until the serve has passed the short line.

(c) On the return of serve, the receiver(s) may not break the plane of the short line, and doing so results in a point for the server.

(d) If the ball bounces on a sideline or the back line on its first bounce, the ball is considered out. When the singles service line is used, a served ball that bounces on it is out. If the ball hits the beveled end of a side wall or the beveled top of the front wall or a side wall and remains in play, the shot is good. A ball that bounces over a side wall is legal; however, local rules may declare that such a shot is out when long-wall courts are used.

(e) Generally, there are no court hinders. Local rules, however, may designate a particular feature of the court as a court hinder. The elements of nature, such as sun, wind, rain, etc., may not serve as the basis for a hinder. A ball that strikes a light pole that is inside the playing area, but outside the "in" zone, without bouncing is considered out. However, if the ball first bounces "in", and then hits such a light pole, it is a court hinder as soon as the ball touches the pole. A court hinder may also be called when a returned ball hits a light attached to the end of a side wall if the ball would have otherwise reached the front wall.

(f) A safety holdup (replay hinder) also includes consideration given to players on an adjacent court or any spectators who are not part of the stationary crowd. The player must be able to hit the ball prior to it reaching the stationary crowd. Any vehicle that enters the playing area can be grounds for a safety holdup. Parked vehicles are classified as part of the stationary crowd.

(g) Intentionally launching a ball following a rally is a technical foul for delay of game against the player who sent the ball sailing. This includes launching a ball prior to the referee or opponent confirming that it is broken.

8.0—Wheelchair

8.1—Changes to Standard Rules

In general, the USAR's standard rules governing racquetball play will be followed, except for the modifications that follow:

(a) Where USAR rules refer to server, person, body, or other similar variations, for wheelchair play such reference shall include all parts of the wheelchair in addition to the person sitting on it.

(b) Where the rules refer to feet, standing or other similar descriptions, for wheelchair play it means only where the rear wheels actually touch the floor.

(c) Where the rules mention body contact, for wheelchair play it shall mean any part of the wheelchair in addition to the player.

(d) Where the rules refer to double bounce or after the first bounce, it shall mean three bounces. All variations of the same phrases shall be revised accordingly.

8.2—Divisions

(a) Novice Division. The Novice Division is for the beginning player who is just learning to play.

(b) Intermediate Division. The Intermediate Division is for the player who has played tournaments before and has a skill level to be competitive in the division.

(c) Open Division. The Open Division is the highest level of play and is for the advanced player.

(d) Multi-bounce Division. The Multi-bounce Division is for the individuals (men or women) whose mobility is such that wheelchair racquetball would be impossible if not for the Multi-bounce Division.

(e) Junior Division. The Junior Divisions are for players who are under the age of 19. The tournament director will determine if the divisions will be played as two-bounce or multi-bounce. Age divisions are: 8–11, 12–15, and 16–18.

8.3—Rules

(a) Two-bounce Rule. Two bounces are used in wheelchair racquetball in all divisions except the Multi-bounce Division. The ball may hit the floor twice before being returned.

(b) Out-of-Chair Rule. The player can neither intentionally jump out of the chair to hit a ball nor stand up in the chair to serve the ball. If the referee determines that the chair was left intentionally, it will result in loss of the rally for the offender. If a player unintentionally leaves the chair, no penalty will be assessed. The referee will warn repeat offenders.

(c) Equipment Standards. To protect playing surfaces, the tournament officials will not allow a person to participate with black tires or anything that will mark or damage the court.

(d) Start. The serve may be started from any place within the service zone. Although the front casters may extend beyond the lines of the service zone, at no time shall the rear wheels cross either the service or short line before the served ball crosses the short line. Penalties for violation are the same as those for the standard game.

(e) Maintenance Delay. A maintenance delay is a delay in the progress of a match due to a malfunction of a wheelchair, prosthesis, or assistive device. Such a delay must be requested by the player and granted by the referee during the match, and shall not exceed five minutes. Only two such delays may be granted for each player for each match. After using both maintenance delays, the player has the following options: (i) continue play with the defective equipment, (ii) immediately substitute replacement equipment, or (iii) postpone the game, with the approval of the referee and opponent.

8.4—Multi-bounce Rules

(a) The ball may bounce as many times as the receiver wants, though the player may swing only once to return the ball to the front wall.

(b) The ball must be hit before it crosses the short line on its way back to the front wall.

(c) The receiver cannot cross the short line after the ball contacts the back wall.

9.0—Visually Impaired

9.1—Eligibility

A player's visual acuity must not be better than 20/200 with the best practical eye correction, or else the player's field of vision must not be better than 20 degrees. The three classifications of blindness are B1 (totally blind to light perception), B2 (able to see hand movement up to 20/600 corrected), and B3 (from 20/600 to 20/200 corrected).

9.2—Return of Serve and Rallies

On the return of serve and on every return thereafter, the player may make multiple attempts to strike the ball until (i) the ball has been touched, (ii) the ball has stopped bouncing, or (iii) the ball has passed the short line after touching the back wall. The only exception is described in Rule 9.3.

9.3—Blast Rule

If the ball (other than on the serve) caroms from the front wall to the back wall on the fly, the player may retrieve the ball from any place on the court—including in front of the short line—so long as the ball has not been touched and is still bouncing.

9.4—Hinders

A replay hinder will result in the rally being replayed without penalty unless the hinder was intentional. If a hinder is clearly intentional, a penalty hinder should be called and the rally awarded to the non-offending player or team.

10.0—Deaf

10.1—Eligibility

An athlete shall have a hearing loss of 55 dB or more in the better ear to be eligible for any tournament for deaf athletes.

11.0—Men's Professional Tour

11.1—Game, Match

All games are played to 11 points, and are won by the player who reaches that score with at least a 2-point lead. If necessary, the game will continue beyond 11 points, until one player has a 2-point lead. Matches are played the best three out of a possible five games.

11.2—Appeals

The referee's call is final. There are no line judges, and no appeals may be made.

11.3—Serve

Players are allowed only one serve to put the ball into play.

11.4—Screen Serve

In IRT matches, screen serves are replayed, except if the serve is also defective for some other reason, such as being long or short.

11.5—Readiness Serve

In IRT matches, any serve made while the opponent is not ready is replayed.

11.6—Court Hinders

No court hinders are allowed or called, except for a wet ball on the first surface—either the floor or side wall—that the serve touches after the front wall.

11.7—Out-of-court Ball

Any ball leaving the court results in a loss of rally.

11.8—Ball

All matches are played with the Penn Pro ball. The first, third, and fifth (if necessary) games of the match are started with a new ball.

11.9—Timeouts

(a) Per Game. Each player is entitled to one 1-minute timeout per game.
(b) Between Points. The player has 10 seconds from the end of the previous rally to put the ball in play.
(c) Between Games. The rest period between all games is two minutes, including between games 4 and 5.
(d) Equipment Timeouts. A player does not have to use regular timeouts to correct or adjust equipment, if the need for the change or adjustment is acknowledged by the referee as being necessary for fair and safe continuation of the match.
(e) Injury Timeout. Consists of two seven and one-half-minute timeouts within a match. Once an injury timeout is taken, the full seven-and-a-half minutes must be used, or it is forfeited.

11.10—Forefeit Time

A match can be forfeited when any player or team fails to report to play 15 minutes after the match was scheduled to be played.

11.11—Apparel

Players must wear collared shirts that are clean and in good repair; however, T-shirts made of some type of performance fabric (Cool Max and Dri-Fit are examples) are acceptable substitutes. Shirts must present a professional appearance and are subject to approval/rejection by the tour commissioner.

12.0—Women's Professional Tour

12.1—Game, Match

Matches are best 3 out of 5 games to 11 points. The first player to score 11 points with at least a 2-point lead wins the game.

12.2—New Ball

A new ball will be used in the first, third, and, if necessary, fifth game.

12.3—Line Judges, Appeals

Line judges are required for semifinal and final matches. Players may use three appeals in each game, plus a game-ending rally may be appealed even if all three appeals have been used.

12.4—Serve

Players are allowed only one serve to put the ball into play.

12.5—Timeouts

(a) Per Game. Each player is entitled to two 45-second timeouts per game. Calling a time-out when none remain will result in a technical foul and deduction of one point from the violator's score.
(b) Between Games. The rest period between all games is one and a half minutes, except between games 4 and 5 when two and a half minutes are allowed.
(c) Wet Court. Player may leave the court to obtain a towel to dry the court, but neither player may leave the court while it is being dried unless she officially calls a timeout.
(d) Equipment Timeouts. Players may only call an equipment timeout if both of her regular timeouts have been exhausted. Equipment must be deemed unsafe to use for an equipment timeout to be called. It cannot be used to change a wet glove. The maximum time allowed for an equipment timeout is 20 seconds.

(e) Injury Timeouts. A total of 15 minutes is allowed for an injury timeout in a match. The injury must be the result of direct contact with the opponent, ball, racquet, wall, or floor. The referee must stop play for any external bleeding so that the player may receive treatment or apply a bandage.

12.6—Hinders

(a) Court Hinders. There are NO court hinders except when the ball strikes a foreign object, including, but not limited to, microphones, speakers, etc. used for production.
(b) Audible Distractions. Audible distractions are NOT a hinder (justification for play stoppage) unless made by the referee during a rally.

13.0—Classic Professional Tour

13.1—Game, Match
Matches are best three out of five games to nine points. Game 5, if necessary, must be won by at least two points and thus may continue beyond nine points.

13.2—Bonus Serve
Players are allowed only one serve, except that once in every game, a player may take a second serve after first advising the referee of his intent.

13.3—Appeals
The referee's call is final. There are no line judges, and no appeals may be made.

13.4—Court Hinders
No court hinders are allowed or called.

14.0—National Masters

14.1—Eligibility
Players at least 45 years of age are eligible to compete in an NMRA event. Competition is offered at five-year age increments. Players must play in their proper age group as determined by their age on the first day of the tournament. You must be a current member of the USAR as of the first and last day of the tournament to compete.

14.2—Draws
All NMRA events are played as round robins. If there are more than 12 players/teams in an age bracket, then it will be split into pools. The top finisher from each pool will play a single elimination playoff to determine the champion. When there are only two flights, the top three players/teams are selected for the playoff. Playoff matches are 2 games to 15 points with a tiebreaker game to 11 (if necessary).

14.3—Game, Match
The number of entrants and available court time dictate the choice of score to win a game, which is usually the first player/team to score either 11 or 15 points. A match consists of two games.

14.4—Match Score
Each player/team receives credit for every point scored during the match. They earn two more points for each game they win, plus an additional four points if they win the match by scoring more overall points than their opponent. However, if each player/team wins a game and the scores are the same, then there is no match winner and the match is recorded as a "tie". A "tie" match results in each player/team earning two points for the game they won, plus two more points, i.e. one half of the four additional points usually earned by the winner of the match.

14.5—Order of Finish
The finishing positions of the players/teams are determined based on who scored the highest average number of points (total overall points earned divided by the total games played).

14.6—Forfeits
If a team/player forfeits a match, they receive zero points for that match and their opponents receive the maximum total points for the match. If a team/player drops out of the tournament, they cannot receive an award. Moreover, the points earned based on the matches they did play are not affected, and the players/teams they did NOT play will have their averages based on the fewer number games they will have played.

Policies and Procedures

A—Tournaments

A.1—Draws
(a) If possible, all draws shall be made at least two days before the tournament commences. The seeding method of drawing shall be approved by the USAR.
(b) At USAR National events, the draw and seeding committee shall be chaired by the USAR's Executive Director, National Tournament Director, and the host tournament director. No other persons shall participate in the draw or seeding unless at the invitation of the draw and seeding committee.
(c) In local and regional tournaments, the draw shall be the responsibility of the tournament director.

A.2—Consolation Matches

(a) Each entrant shall be entitled to participate in a minimum of two matches. Therefore, losers of their first match shall have the opportunity to compete in a consolation bracket of their own division. In draws of less than seven players, a round robin may be offered. See A.6 about how to determine the winner of a round robin event.

(b) Consolation matches may be waived at the discretion of the tournament director, but this waiver must be in writing on the tournament application.

(c) Preliminary consolation matches will be 2 of 3 games to 11 points. Semifinal and final matches will follow the regular scoring format.

A.3—Scheduling

(a) Preliminary Matches. If contestants are entered in more than one division, it is likely that they will be required to play several times on the same day with little rest between matches. This is a risk assumed on entering multiple categories of play. If possible, schedules should provide at least one hour of rest between matches.

(b) Final Matches. Where the possibility exists of one or more players reaching the finals in multiple divisions, it is recommended that these matches be scheduled several hours apart to assure more rest between the final matches. If this is not possible, it is recommended that a singles final be scheduled before any doubles final, and that at least one hour of rest be llowed between matches.

(c) Conflicts. If a player reaches the finals of two divisions that are scheduled within the same hour, that player should be given the option of choosing which final is to be played first.

A.4—Notice of Matches

After the first round of matches, it is the responsibility of each player to check the posted schedules to determine the time and place of each subsequent match. If any change is made in the schedule after posting, it shall be the duty of the tournament director to notify the players of the change.

A.5—Finishes

Finalists must play off for first and second place, or determine a winner by some mutually acceptable method. Semifinalists are not required to play off for third place. However, if one semifinalist wishes to play off and the other does not, the one willing to play shall be awarded third place.

A.6—Round Robin Scoring

The final positions of players or teams in round robin competition is determined by the following sequence:

(a) Winner of the most matches;

(b) In a two-way tie, winner of the head-to-head match;

(c) In a tie of three or more, the first tiebreaker is the net difference between the numbers of games that each of those players won and lost when they played each other. Matches played against persons NOT involved in the tie are NOT counted. The player with the largest positive difference is awarded the position in question.

 1. If a two-way tie remains, the winner of the head-to-head match is awarded the higher position.

 2. If a multiple tie remains, the second tiebreaker is the net difference between the numbers of points that each player won and lost when they played each other. Matches played against persons NOT involved in the tie are NOT counted. The player with the largest positive difference is awarded the position in question.

 3. If a multiple tie still remains, the player who scored the highest average points per match is awarded the position in question. Matches played against persons NOT involved in the tie are NOT counted.

A.7—Court Assignments

In all USAR-sanctioned tournaments, the tournament director and/or USAR official in attendance may decide on a change of court after the completion of any tournament game, if such a change will accommodate better spectator conditions.

A.8—Warm-up Times

Once all players in a match have been informed what court they will be playing on, singles players are allowed up to five minutes of on-court warm-up time, and these warm-up times run concurrently. For doubles, each team is allowed up to five minutes for on-court warm-up, and while these times do not run concurrently, both teams' warm-ups must be completed generally within a 10-minute period that starts when the first team begins its warm-up.

A.9—Tournament Conduct

In all USAR sanctioned tournaments, the referee is empowered to forfeit a match, if the conduct of a player or team is considered detrimental to the tournament and the game. See B.5(d) and (e).

A.10—Spectator Conduct

In the event of disruptive or threatening behavior on the part of any spectator, relative, parent, guardian, or coach at any USAR-sanctioned event, the referee is empowered to address a first offense by enforcing Sanction 1 detailed below. For additional infractions, the tournament director, or USAR official in attendance, either of their own accord or at the request of the referee, is empowered to enforce Sanctions 2 and 3 as warranted.

1. For the first offense: violator may watch, but not speak, while the athlete's match is being played.
2. For the second offense: violator may not watch the athlete's match, but may remain within the building.
3. For the third offense: violator will be removed from the club for the duration of the tournament, and pertinent authorities advised of the restriction. If a given situation so warrants, the tournament director or USAR official may invoke this sanction immediately and without previous offenses—in the interest of safety.

B—Officiating

B.1—Tournament Management

All USAR-sanctioned tournaments shall be managed by a tournament director, who shall designate the officials.

B.2—Rules Committee

The tournament director should appoint a tournament rules committee to resolve any disputes that the referee, tournament desk, or tournament director cannot resolve. The committee, composed of an odd number of persons, may include state or national officials, or other qualified individuals in attendance that are prepared to meet on short notice. The tournament director should not be a member of this committee.

B.3—Referee Appointment and Removal

The principal official for every match shall be the referee who has been designated by the tournament director, or a designated representative, and who has been agreed upon by all participants in the match. The referee's authority regarding a match begins once the players are called to the court. The referee may be removed from a match upon the agreement of all participants (teams in doubles) or at the discretion of the tournament director or the designated representative. In the event that a referee's removal is requested by one player or team and not agreed to by the other, the tournament director or the designated representative may accept or reject the request. It is suggested that the match be observed before determining what, if any, action is to be taken. In addition, two line judges and a scorekeeper may also be designated to assist the referee in officiating the match.

B.4—Rules Briefing

Before all tournaments, all officials and players shall be briefed on rules as well as local court hinders, regulations, and modifications the tournament director wishes to impose. The briefing should be reduced to writing. The current USAR rules will apply and be made available. Any modifications the tournament director wishes to impose must be stated on the entry form and be available to all players at registration.

B.5—Referees

(a) Pre-match Duties. Before each match begins, it shall be the duty of the referee to:

1. Check on adequacy of preparation of court with respect to cleanliness, lighting, and temperature.
2. Check on availability and suitability of materials to include balls, towels, scorecards, pencils, and timepiece necessary for the match.
3. Check the readiness and qualifications of the line judges and scorekeeper. Review appeal procedures and instruct them of their duties, rules, and local regulations.
4. Go onto the court to make introductions; brief the players on court hinders (both designated and undesignated); identify any out-of-play areas [see Rule 2.1(a)]; discuss local regulations and rule modifications for this tournament; and explain often-misinterpreted rules.
5. Inspect players' equipment; identify the line judges; verify selection of a primary and alternate ball.
6. Toss coin and offer the winner the choice of serving or receiving.

(b) Decisions. During the match, the referee shall make all decisions with regard to the rules. Where line judges are used, the referee shall announce all final judgments. If both players in singles and three out of four in a doubles match disagree with a call made by the referee, the referee is overruled, with the exception of technical fouls and forfeitures.

(c) Protests. Any decision not involving the judgment of the referee will, on protest, be accorded due process as set forth in the constitution of the USAR. For the purposes of rendering a prompt decision regarding protests filed during the course of an ongoing tournament, the stages of due process will be: first to the tournament desk, then to the tournament director, and finally to the tournament rules committee. In those instances when time permits, the protest may be elevated to the state association or, when appropriate, to the national level as called for in the USAR constitution.

(d) Forfeitures. A match may be forfeited by the referee when:

1. Any player refuses to abide by the referee's decision or engages in unsportsmanlike conduct.

2. Any player or team who fails to report to play 10 minutes after the match has been scheduled to play. (The tournament director may permit a longer delay if circumstances warrant such a decision.)

3. A game will be forfeited by the referee for using an illegal racquet as specified in Rule 2.4(e).

(e) Defaults. A player or team may be forfeited by the tournament director or official for failure to comply with the tournament or host facility's rules while on the premises between matches, or for abuse of hospitality, locker room, or other rules and procedures.

(f) Spectators. The referee shall have jurisdiction over the spectators, as well as the players, while the match is in progress.

(g) Other Rulings. The referee may rule on all matters not covered in the USAR Official Rules. However, the referee's ruling is subject to protest as described in B.5(c).

B.6—Line Judges

(a) When Utilized. Two line judges should be used for semifinal and final matches, when requested by a player or team, or when the referee or tournament director so desires. However, the use of line judges is subject to availability and the discretion of the tournament director.

(b) Replacing Line Judges. If any player objects to a person serving as a line judge before the match begins, all reasonable effort shall be made to find a replacement acceptable to the officials and players. If a player objects after the match begins, any replacement shall be at the discretion of the referee and/or tournament director.

(c) Position of Line Judges. The players and referee shall designate the court location of the line judges. The tournament director shall settle any dispute.

(d) Duties and Responsibilities. Line judges are designated to help decide appeals. In the event of an appeal, and after a very brief explanation of the appeal by the referee, the line judges must indicate their opinion of the referee's call.

(e) Signals. Line judges should extend their arm and signal as follows: (i) thumb up to show agreement with the referee's call, (ii) thumb down to show disagreement, and (iii) hand open with palm facing down to indicate "no opinion" or that the play in question wasn't seen.

(f) Manner of Response. Line judges should be careful not to signal until the referee announces the appeal and asks for a ruling. In responding to the referee's request, line judges should not look at each other, but indicate their opinions simultaneously in clear view of the players and referee. If at any time a line judge is unsure of which call is being appealed or what the referee's call was, the line judge should ask the referee to repeat the call and the appeal.

(g) Result of Response. The referee's call stands if at least one line judge agrees with the referee or if neither line judge has an opinion. If both line judges disagree with the referee, the referee must reverse the call. If one line judge disagrees with the referee and the other signals no opinion, the rally is replayed. Any replays, with the exception of appeals on the second serve itself, will result in resumption of play at first serve.

B.7—Appeals

(a) Appealable Calls and Non-calls. In any match using line judges, a player may appeal any call or non-call by the referee, except for a technical foul or forfeiture.

(b) How to Appeal. A verbal appeal by a player must be made directly to the referee immediately after the rally has ended. A player who believes there is an infraction to appeal should bring it to the attention of the referee and line judges by raising the non-racquet hand at the time the perceived infraction occurs. The player is obligated to continue to play until the rally has ended or the referee stops play. The referee will recognize a player's appeal only if it is made before that player leaves the court for any reason including timeouts and game-ending rallies or, if that player doesn't leave the court, before the next serve begins.

(c) Loss of Appeal. A player or team forfeits its right of appeal for that rally if the appeal is made directly to the line judges or if the appeal is made after an excessive demonstration or complaint.

(d) Limit on Appeals. A player or team can make three appeals per game. However, if either line judge disagrees (thumb down) with the referee's call, that appeal will not count against the three-appeal limit. In addition, a potential game-ending rally may be appealed without charge against the limit—even if the three-appeal limit has been reached.

B.8—Outcome of Appeals

Everything except technical fouls and forfeitures can be appealed. The following outcomes cover several of the most common types of appeal, but not all possible appeals could be addressed. Therefore, referee's discretion and common sense should govern the outcomes of those appeals that are not covered herein:

(a) Skip Ball. If the referee makes a call of "skip ball," and the call is reversed, the referee then must decide if the shot in question could have been returned had play continued. If, in the opinion of the referee, the shot could have been returned, the rally shall be replayed. However, if the shot was not retrievable, the side that hit the shot in question is declared the winner of the rally. If the referee makes no call on a shot (thereby indicating that the shot did not skip), an appeal may be made that the shot skipped. If the "no call" is reversed, the side that hit the shot in question loses the rally.

(b) Fault Serve. If the referee makes a call of fault serve and the call is reversed, the serve is re-played—unless the referee considered the serve to have been irretrievable, in which case a point is awarded to the server. If an appeal is made because the referee makes no call on a serve (thereby indicating that the serve was good) and the "no call" is reversed, the result will be a fault serve.

(c) Out Serve. If the referee calls an "out serve" and the call is reversed, the serve will be replayed, unless the serve was obviously a fault too, in which case the call becomes fault serve. However, if the call is reversed and the serve was considered an ace, a point will be awarded. Also, if the referee makes no call on a serve—thereby indicating that the serve was good—but the "no call" is reversed, it results in an immediate loss of serve.

(d) Double Bounce Pickup. If the referee makes a call of two bounces, and the call is reversed, the rally is replayed, except if the player against whom the call was made hit a shot that could not have been retrieved; then that player wins the rally. (Before awarding a rally in this situation, the referee must be certain that the shot would not have been retrieved even if play had not been halted.) If an appeal is made because the referee makes no call, thereby indicating that the get was not two bounces, and the "no call" is reversed, the player who made the two-bounce pickup is declared the loser of the rally.

(e) Receiving Line Violation (Encroachment). If the referee makes a call of encroachment, but the call is overturned, the serve shall be replayed unless the return was deemed irretrievable, in which case a sideout (or possibly a handout in doubles) should be called. When an appeal is made because the referee made no call, and the appeal is successful, the server is awarded a point.

(f) Court Hinder. If the referee makes a call of court hinder during a rally or return of serve, the rally is replayed. If the referee makes no call and a player feels that a court hinder occurred, that player may appeal. If the appeal is successful, the rally will be replayed. If a court hinder occurs on a second serve, play resumes at second serve.

B.9—Rule Interpretations

If a player feels the referee has interpreted the rules incorrectly, the player may require the referee or tournament director to cite the applicable rule in the rulebook. Having discovered a misapplication or misinterpretation, the official must correct the error by replaying the rally, awarding the point, calling "Sideout," or taking other corrective measures.

C—Eligibility and National Events

C.1—Eligibility

To be eligible to compete in any USAR-sanctioned event, a player must only be a valid, registered member of USA Racquetball.

C.2—Waiver & Release

Athletic Waiver and Release of Liability: In consideration of being allowed to participate in any USA Racquetball athletics/sports programs, and related events and activities, all member signatories:

1. Agree that prior to participating, they will inspect the facilities and equipment to be used, and if they believe anything is unsafe, they will immediately advise their coach, supervisor, or USAR personnel of such condition(s) and refuse to participate.

2. Acknowledge and fully understand that each participant will be engaging in activities that involve risk of serious injury, including permanent disability and death, and severe social

and economic losses which might result not only from their own actions, inaction, or negligence but the actions, inaction, or negligence of others, the rules of play, or the condition of the premises or of any equipment used. Further, that there may be other risks not known to us or not reasonably foreseeable at this time.

3. Assume all the foregoing risks and accept personal responsibility for the damages following such injury, permanent disability, or death.

4. Release, waive, discharge, and covenant not to sue USA Racquetball; its affiliated Clubs; regional sports organizations; their respective administrators, directors, agents, coaches, and other employees of the organization; other participants; sponsoring agencies, sponsors, advertisers; and, if applicable, owners and lessees of premises used to conduct the event, all of which are hereinafter referred to as "releases" from any and all liability to the signatory on the opposite side of this form, his or her heirs and next of kin for any and all claims, demands, losses or damages on account of injury including death or damage to property, caused or alleged to be caused in whole or in part by the negligence of the release or otherwise.

C.3—Recognized Divisions

Title opportunities at national championships will be selected from the division lists that follow. Combined Age and Skill Divisions may also be offered to provide additional competitive opportunities for non-open entrants. For ranking consistency, state organizations are encouraged to select from these recognized divisions when establishing competition in all sanctioned events:

(a) Open Division. Any eligible player, as defined in C.1.

(b) Adult Age Divisions. Eligibility is determined by the player's age on the first day of the tournament that anyone begins playing in that division. Divisions are:

- 24 & under _____ Varsity
- 25+ _____ Junior Veterans
- 30+ _____ Veterans
- 35+ _____ Seniors
- 40+ _____ Veteran Seniors
- 45+ _____ Masters
- 50+ _____ Veteran Masters
- 55+ _____ Golden Masters
- 60+ _____ Veteran Golden Masters
- 65+ _____ Senior Golden Masters
- 70+ _____ Advanced Golden Masters
- 75+ _____ Super Golden Masters
- 80+ _____ Grand Masters
- 85+ _____ Super Grand Masters

(c) Junior Age Divisions. Player eligibility is determined by the player's age on January 1st of the current calendar year. Divisions are:

- 18 & Under
- 16 & Under
- 14 & Under
- 12 & Under
- 10 & Under
- 8 & Under (regular rules)
- 8 & Under (multi-bounce rules)
- 6 & Under (multi-bounce rules)

(d) Skill Divisions. Player eligibility is determined by AmPRO skill level certification or verification by a state association official, at the entered level:

- Elite [Open level drop-down]
- A
- B
- C
- D
- Novice

(e) Age and Skill Divisions. Player eligibility is determined by the player's age on the first day of the tournament, plus AmPRO skill level certification, or verification by a state association official, at the entered level. Such combinations may be offered as additional competition to players who do not fall into the "open" or designated skill levels of play. For example: 24- A/B; 30+ B; 35+ C/D; 40+ A; 65+ A/B, etc.

C.4—Competion By Gender

Men and women may compete only in events and divisions for their respective gender during regional and national tournaments. If there is not sufficient number of players to warrant play in a specific division, the tournament director may place the entrants in a comparably competitive division. Note: For the purpose of encouraging the development of women's racquetball, the governing bodies of numerous states permit women to play in men's divisions when a comparable skill level is not available in the women's divisions.

C.5—USAR Regional Championships

(a) Adult Regional Tournaments

1. Regional tournaments will be conducted at various metropolitan sites designated annually by the USAR and players may compete at any site they choose.

2. A person may compete in any number of adult regional tournaments, but may not enter a championship division (as listed in C.4) after having won that division at a previous adult regional tournament that same year.

3. A person cannot participate in more than two championship events at a regional tournament.

4. Any awards or remuneration to a USAR National Championship will be posted on the entry blank.

(b) Junior Regional Tournaments. Certain regions still host regional qualifying events. Qualification for Junior Nationals is either the regionals or state championships.

C.6—U.S. National Singles and Doubles Championships

The U.S. National Singles and Doubles Tournaments are separate tournaments and are played on different dates. National Singles are traditionally held in May; National Doubles are held in February.

(a) Competition in an Adult Regional singles tournament (or recognized qualifying event) is required to qualify for the National Singles Championship. Recognized qualifying events are:
- WSMA Championships (January)
- NMRA Singles Championships (February)
- World Intercollegiate Championships (April)
- individual state championships.

(b) The National Tournament Director may handle the rating of each region and determine how many players shall qualify from each regional tournament.

C.7—U.S. National Junior Olympic Championships

It will be conducted on a different date than all other National Championships. Traditionally held in June.

C.8—U.S. National High School Championships

It will be conducted on a different date than all other National Championships. Traditionally held in March.

C.9—IRF World Intercollegiate Championships

It will be conducted on a different date than all other National Championships. Traditionally held in April.

C.10—U.S. Open Racquetball Championships

It will be conducted on a different date than all other National Championships, and include both pro and USAR competitive divisions.

D—Procedures

D.1—Rule Change Procedures

To ensure the orderly growth of racquetball, the USAR has established specific procedures that are followed before a major change is made to the rules of the game.

NOTE: Changes to rules and regulations in Sections 1 through 10 must adhere to published rule change procedures. Remaining sections may be altered by vote of the USAR Board of Directors*.

(a) Rule change proposals must be submitted in writing to the USAR National Office by June 1st.

(b) The USAR Board of Directors will review all proposals at its Fall board meeting and determine which will be considered.

(c) Selected proposals will appear in RACQUETBALL Magazine—the official USAR publication—as soon as possible after the Fall board meeting for comment by the general membership.

(d) After reviewing membership input and the recommendations of the National Rules Committee and National Rules Commissioner, the proposals are discussed and voted upon at the annual Board of Directors meeting in May.

(e) Changes approved in May become effective on September 1st. Exception: changes in racquet specifications become effective 2 years later on September 1st.

(f) Proposed rules that are considered for adoption in one year, but are not approved by the Board of Directors in May of that year, will not be considered for adoption the following year.

* The following policies and procedures segments are subject to stated rule change procedures outlined in D.1:
- A.6 Round Robin Scoring
- A.8 Tournament Conduct
- B.5 (d–g) Forfeitures, Defaults …
- B.6 Line Judges
- B.7 Appeals
- B.8 Outcome of Appeals

D.2—National Rules Commissioner

Otto Dietrich, National Rules Commissioner
4244 Russet Court
Lilburn, GA 30047-3346
770-972-2303
(Office/Home)
678-575-8975 (Cell)
Email: ODietrich@USRA.org

Answer Key to Checkpoints

Chapter 1
1. c 2. b 3. d 4. d 5. d 6. d 7. b 8. b

Chapter 2
1. a 2. a 3. c 4. d 5. b 6. b 7. c 8. a

Chapter 3
1. a 2. b 3. d 4. b 5. a 6. b 7. d 8. b

Chapter 4
1. a 2. b 3. a 4. b 5. c 6. b 7. a 8. c

Chapter 5
1. b 2. d 3. d 4. d 5. c 6. a 7. d 8. c

Chapter 6
1. c 2. b 3. d 4. d 5. c 6. b 7. a 8. c

Chapter 7
1. d 2. d 3. a 4. b 5. a 6. b 7. c 8. d

Chapter 8
1. a 2. d 3. a 4. d 5. d 6. d 7. b 8. c
9. a 10. d

Chapter 9
1. d 2. d 3. a 4. b 5. a 6. d 7. e 8. e 9. b
10. d 11. e 12. b 13. d

Chapter 10
None

Chapter 11
1. a 2. d 3. b 4. a 5. a 6. a 7. c 8. d

Photo Credits

Chapter One
p. 1 Photography by Terrell Lloyd; assisted by Greg Harris and Tim May; p. 3 Photography by J. E. Bryant; p. 4 Photography by J. E. Bryant; p. 5 Photography by J. E. Bryant; p. 6 (top) Photography by J. E. Bryant, (center) Photography by Eric Risberg, (bottom) Photography by Terrell Lloyd; assisted by Greg Harris and Tim May; p. 7 Photography by Terrell Lloyd; assisted by Greg Harris and Tim May

Chapter Two
p. 11 Photography by Terrell Lloyd; assisted by Greg Harris and Tim May; p. 16 Photography by Terrell Lloyd; assisted by Greg Harris and Tim May; p. 17 Photography by Terrell Lloyd; assisted by Greg Harris and Tim May; p. 18 Photography by Terrell Lloyd; assisted by Greg Harris and Tim May; p. 19 Photography by Terrell Lloyd; assisted by Greg Harris and Tim May; p. 20 Photography by Terrell Lloyd; assisted by Greg Harris and Tim May

Chapter Three
p. 23 Photography by Terrell Lloyd; assisted by Greg Harris and Tim May; p. 24 (top left) Photography by Eric Risberg, (top center) Photography by Greg Hazard, (center) Photography by Greg Hazard, (bottom left) Photography by Eric Risberg, (bottom right) Photography by Eric Risberg; p. 25 (top) Photography by Eric Risberg, (bottom) Photography by Greg Hazard; p. 26 Photography by Eric Risberg; p. 27 Photography by Terrell Lloyd; assisted by Greg Harris and Tim May; p. 28 (left, right) Photography by Terrell Lloyd; assisted by Greg Harris and Tim May, (inset) Photo by Eric Risberg; p. 29 Photography by Terrell Lloyd; assisted by Greg Harris and Tim May; p. 30 Photography by Terrell Lloyd; assisted by Greg Harris and Tim May; p. 31 Photography by Terrell Lloyd; assisted by Greg Harris and Tim May; p. 32 Photography by Terrell Lloyd; assisted by Greg Harris and Tim May; p. 33 Photography by Terrell Lloyd; assisted by Greg Harris and Tim May, (inset) Photo by Greg Hazard; p. 34 Photography by Terrell Lloyd; assisted by Greg Harris and Tim May; p. 35 Photography by Terrell Lloyd; assisted by Greg Harris and Tim May; p. 36 Photography by Terrell Lloyd; assisted by Greg Harris and Tim May

Chapter Four
p. 39 Photography by Terrell Lloyd; assisted by Greg Harris and Tim May; p. 40 (top right) Photography by Terrell Lloyd; assisted by Greg Harris and Tim May, (top right inset) Photo by Eric Risberg, (center) Photography by Terrell Lloyd; assisted by Greg Harris and Tim May, (center inset) Photo by Greg Hazard, (bottom two rows) Photography by Terrell Lloyd; assisted by Greg Harris and Tim May; p. 41 Photography by Terrell Lloyd; assisted by Greg Harris and Tim May; p. 42 Photography by Terrell Lloyd; assisted by Greg Harris and Tim May; p. 43 Photography by Terrell Lloyd; assisted by Greg Harris and Tim May; p. 44 Photography by Terrell Lloyd; assisted by Greg Harris and Tim May, (inset) Photo by Eric Risberg; p. 46 Photography by Terrell Lloyd; assisted by Greg Harris and Tim May; p. 47 Photography by Terrell Lloyd; assisted by Greg Harris and Tim May

Chapter Five
p. 51 Photography by Terrell Lloyd; assisted by Greg Harris and Tim May; p. 52 Photography by Terrell Lloyd; assisted by Greg Harris and Tim May, (inset) Photo by Eric Risberg; p. 53 Photography by Terrell Lloyd; assisted by Greg Harris and Tim May, (top inset) Photo by Greg Hazard, (center inset) Photo by Eric Risberg; p. 55 Photography by Terrell Lloyd; assisted by Greg Harris and Tim May, (inset) Photo by Greg Hazard

Chapter Six
p. 61 Photography by Terrell Lloyd; assisted by Greg Harris and Tim May; p. 62 Photography by Terrell Lloyd; assisted by Greg Harris and Tim May; p. 63 Photography by Terrell Lloyd; assisted by Greg Harris and Tim May; p. 64 Photography by Terrell Lloyd; assisted by Greg Harris and Tim May, (inset) Photo by Eric Risberg; p. 67 Photography by Terrell Lloyd; assisted by Greg Harris and Tim May, (inset) Photo by Greg Hazard

Chapter Seven
p. 71 Photography by Terrell Lloyd; assisted by Greg Harris and Tim May; p. 72 Photography by Terrell Lloyd; assisted by Greg Harris and Tim May; p. 74 Photography by Terrell Lloyd; assisted by Greg Harris and Tim May; p. 76 Photography by Terrell Lloyd; assisted by Greg Harris and Tim May

Chapter Eight
p. 79 Photography by Terrell Lloyd; assisted by Greg Harris and Tim May; p. 80 Photography by Terrell Lloyd; assisted by Greg Harris and Tim May; p. 81 Photography by Terrell Lloyd; assisted by Greg Harris and Tim May; p. 82 Photography by Terrell Lloyd; assisted by Greg Harris and Tim May; p. 83 Photography by Terrell Lloyd; assisted by Greg Harris and Tim May

Chapter Nine
p. 87 Photography by Terrell Lloyd; assisted by Greg Harris and Tim May; p. 88 Photography by Terrell Lloyd; assisted by Greg Harris and Tim May; p. 89 Photography by Terrell Lloyd; assisted by Greg Harris and Tim May

Chapter Ten
p. 97 Photography by Terrell Lloyd; assisted by Greg Harris and Tim May; p. 99 Photography by Terrell Lloyd; assisted by Greg Harris and Tim May; p. 106 Photography by Terrell Lloyd; assisted by Greg Harris and Tim May

Chapter Eleven
p. 105 Photography by Terrell Lloyd; assisted by Greg Harris and Tim May; p. 108 Photography by Terrell Lloyd; assisted by Greg Harris and Tim May; p. 109 Photography by Terrell Lloyd; assisted by Greg Harris and Tim May; p. 110 Photography by Terrell Lloyd; assisted by Greg Harris and Tim May; p. 111 Photography by Terrell Lloyd; assisted by Greg Harris and Tim May; p. 112 (top center) Photography by J. E. Bryant, (center) Photography by J. E. Bryant, (bottom left, center) Photography by Terrell Lloyd; assisted by Greg Harris and Tim May; p. 113 Photography by Terrell Lloyd; assisted by Greg Harris and Tim May; p. 114 (top) Photography by Eric Risberg, (center) Photography by Terrell Lloyd; assisted by Greg Harris and Tim May; p. 117 Photography by Terrell Lloyd; assisted by Greg Harris and Tim May; p. 120 Photo by J. E. Bryant

Glossary of Terms

Ace: A legal serve that the receiver of the serve totally missed.

Aerobic: Exercise that does not create an oxygen debt.

Aerobic conditioning: Conditioning program that emphasizes efficient utilization of oxygen in order to recover quickly.

Alley: The lane along the side walls that is a target for down-the-line passing shots.

Anaerobic metabolism: The release of energy without the use of oxygen.

Around-the-wall ball: A defensive shot that hits three walls before touching the floor.

Back court: That section of the court nearest the back wall and described as the last third of the court.

Backhand: A stroke hit from the non-racquet side of the body.

Backswing: The preparation phase of the basic swing.

Back wall: The rear wall, usually the entrance to the court area.

Blocking: A penalty hinder in which an opponent assumes a position on court that eliminates a fair opportunity for the other player.

Ceiling–front wall shot: A defensive shot that strikes the ceiling and front wall.

Ceiling shot: A ball that strikes ceiling–front wall in sequence.

Center court: The area immediately behind the short line and equal distance from the side walls.

Center-court position: The most strategically advantageous area for a player to be positioned.

Closed face: Position of the racquet face on the ball when hitting the ball downward (usually turned away from the ceiling).

Continental grip: The grip positioned halfway between the Eastern forehand and the backhand grip.

Corner kill shot: A kill shot that strikes the front wall–side wall and rebounds into the direction of mid-court.

Corner shot or corner shot return: A ball that strikes the back and side wall simultaneously and is returned off the rebound of these two walls.

Cross-court pass: A two-wall passing shot executed when the opponent is either on the same side as you or is in an "up" position. The ball hits the front wall and then the side wall.

Court position: Position a player assumes in order to be effective on the next shot.

Crotch shot: A ball simultaneously striking two playing surfaces (such as wall and floor).

Cut-throat: A three-player racquetball game designed with the server playing against the other two players.

Defensive shots: Shots that prevent the opponent from holding an offensive court position.

Dehydration: Condition brought on by loss of body fluids.

Doubles: A four-player racquetball game played between teams of two players.

Down-the-line pass: A shot that carries along a side wall one to two feet from the wall and below the opponent's waist. This also is called down-the-wall and it is designed to pass an opponent who is in an "up" position.

Drive: A powerfully hit shot that follows a straight path off the front wall.

Drive serve: A powerfully hit serve that follows a straight path off the front wall.

Drive serve zone: The zone defined by two lines 3 feet from each side wall in the service box that divides the service zone into two 17-foot service zones for drive serves. The zone is associated with the special rule regarding drive serves.

Drop shot: A touch shot that is hit with deception and little force.

Eastern backhand grip: The conventional backhand grip that is assumed by rotating the racquet a quarter turn to the racquet side of the body from the Eastern forehand grip.

Eastern forehand grip: The conventional racquetball grip best described as a "shakehands" position.

Endurance: Ability to maintain power for extended period.

Exercise heart rate: The heart rate measured as 70–80 percent of a maximal heart rate.

Fault: A serve that touches the floor before passing the short line, or one in which the ball strikes the front wall and the ceiling, the back wall, or two side walls before hitting the floor. These serves are illegal and must be replayed. Two faults result in a sideout.

Fault serves: Any serve that by rule results in an out.

Flexibility: Ease and range of movement.

Follow-through: Arm movement after hitting the ball.

Foot fault: An illegal serve identified by the server's foot touching the outside of the service area, or in doubles when the server's partner is not positioned in the service box during the serve.

Forehand: A stroke hit from the racquet side of the body.

Foreward swing: Hitting the ball with force directed toward the front wall.

Front court: That section of the court in front of the service line.

Front-wall kill: A kill shot that hits the front wall straight on and rebounds toward the back wall without touching a side wall.

Front-wall–straight-in kill shot: A kill shot that strikes the front wall first and then rebounds toward the back wall without touching a side wall.

Garbage serve: A serve hit between the speed of a drive and a lob serve that bounces between the shoulder and waist to the receiver. The serve gives an illusion of a mishit serve.

Grip: Position of the hand on the racquet.

Handout: Change of serves in doubles.

Heatstroke: A medical condition caused by prolonged hyperthermia.

High-Z serve: A serve that strikes high off the front wall (near the ceiling) and follows a "Z" pattern across the court.

Hinder: Any situation that prevents an opponent from having a fair shot at hitting the ball during a rally. Hinders include penalty and replay hinders.

Hyperthermia: Elevated body temperature.

Kill shot: Any ball that strikes the front wall hard and low so the rebound with the floor occurs almost simultaneously with the wall. A winning offensive shot.

Legal serve: A serve that strikes the front wall and no more than one side wall before passing the short line and striking the floor.

Lob: A defensive shot, hit along a side wall so it follows a path high over center court and falls with little rebound into a back corner. This ball may touch a side wall close to the back corner.

Lob serve: A serve hit high off the front wall that lands deep in the back court.

Long: A serve that strikes the back wall on the fly. A fault.

Long-bodies: An extra extra-length racquet.

Low-Z serve: A power serve striking front and side wall and opposite back corner.

Match: The culmination of a competition with the winner usually winning two of three games. The first two games are played to 15 points; the third game, if required, is played to 11 points.

Maximal heart rate: Maximum speed the heart can beat during exercise.

Midcourt: The area between the service and short line and the two side walls.

Muscular endurance: Helps to maintain power during long rallies or through a prolonged match.

Muscular strength: This is in reference to the degree of strength of the muscles that provide power to the various power shots in racquetball (i.e., muscular strength concentrated on the arms, shoulders, chest, upper back, abdominals, and legs).

Non-thinking strategy: Following a defensive reactive strategy with few decisions to make.

Offensive shot: The attempt to win a point outright by virtue of the skill with which the shot is hit.

On edge: The position of the racquet face when it is perpendicular to the floor.

One-wall racquetball: Racquetball played with front wall only.

Open-face: Position of the racquet face on the ball when hitting the ball up (usually turned toward the ceiling).

Out: End of a point.

Out serves: Serves including non-front-wall serve, touched serve, crotch serve, illegal hit, out-of-order serve, safety zone violation, or fake serve, all resulting in loss of serve.

Overhead: Shots hit from above-the-shoulder position with an extended arm.

Overhead kill shot: A kill shot hit off a ball positioned above the shoulder.

Over-the-shoulder: A ball hit from a position directly over the shoulder.

Passing shot: An offensive shot that literally goes past an opponent who is in the front-, mid-, or center-court positions.

Penalty hinder: Interference with the opponent's opportunity to play a shot fairly, including failure to move, stroke interference, blocking, moving into the ball, pushing, intentional distractions, obstruction of view, and wetting of the ball.

Pinch kill shot: A shot that strikes the side wall–front wall sequence and that is unreturnable because of the low position, high velocity of the shot. Also called a pinch shot.

Pivot: Turning to the side in order to hit the ball.

Protective eyewear: Safety glasses required for wear when entering a racquetball court.

Racquet face: The portion of the racquet with which the ball is struck during play.

Rally: An alternating, continuous exchange of shots during the play of a point.

Receiver: Player who receives the serve.

Receiving line: The line identified by the intermittent floor marks located five feet behind the short line. A player may not stand in front of the receiving line to receive a serve.

Replay hinder: An unintentional interference with the opponent's opportunity to play a shot fairly, including: court hinders, ball hitting an opponent, body contact, screen ball, backswing hinder, and a safety holdup.

Roll-out: A perfect kill shot defined by the action of the ball striking the front wall and rolling on the floor with no bounce.

Run-the-corner: A ball that rebounds to a back corner, hitting the side wall and back wall before striking the floor.

Safety hinder: When an opponent stops play to avoid contact with the other player that could result in injury.

Safety zone: The five-foot area defined by the area between the back edge of the short line and the receiving line. During the process of the serve, the receiver must wait for the ball to either bounce or cross the short line before stepping into the safety zone to return the serve.

Screen: A blocking of the opponent's vision, preventing the opponent from seeing the ball.

Service box: The 18-inch box at each end of the service area where, in doubles, the server's partner stands until a legal serve has been executed by crossing the short line.

Service line: The line on the floor closest to the front wall. The front line of the service zone.

Service return: The shot hit in response to the serve at the beginning of each point.

Service zone: The area between the service line and the short line. The area of the court for the server to legally execute the serve.

Serving: Placing ball in play.

Set: The ready position. The position that enables the receiver of a shot to turn or pivot to hit the ball.

Setup: An easy shot that should be converted into an easy scoring opportunity for the hitter.

Short: A served ball that touches the floor in front of or on the short line. A fault.

Short line: The back line of the service zone positioned 20 feet from the front wall. For a serve to be legal, it must rebound past this line.

Side wall: Two walls that are perpendicular to the front and back walls.

Sideout: Loss of a serve to the opponent.

Skip ball: A shot that hits the floor before reaching the front wall. Usually a skip close to the front wall is difficult to determine.

Sportsmanship ethic: An attitude of fair play.

Tether: The safety strap attached to the racquet grip and secured around the racquet wrist area. Also called a thong.

Thinking strategy: The act of taking advantage of an opponent through the use of intellect, court strategy, and skill.

Three-wall racquetball: An alternative playing surface and court configuration minus a back wall and ceiling. With adaptation, games of singles, doubles, and cut-throat are played just as on a regulation four-wall court.

Three-wall shot: A defensive shot that rebounds off three walls.

Volley: Striking the ball in midair from a rebound off the front wall before the ball touches the floor.

Wallpaper shot: A ball that rebounds along a side wall, making a return extremely difficult.

Warm-up: Exercise engaged in before play that helps to prepare the body for activity.

Western grip: A grip that is used for a forehand stroke. It is similar to the grip used on a racquet when it is picked up off the floor.

Wrist cock: Position of the wrist that allows a "snapping" action at contact with the ball.

Z serve: A ball hit at shoulder height that strikes the front and side wall simultaneously and then hits the opposite back corner.

Index